Atlas of Sectional Radiological Anatomy for PET/CT

Mehmet T. Kitapçı

Atlas of Sectional Radiological Anatomy for PET/CT

Springer

Mehmet T. Kitapçı, M.D.
Department of Nuclear Medicine
Gazi University School of Medicine
Ankara, Turkey
kitapci@gazi.edu.tr

ISBN 978-1-4614-1526-8 ISBN 978-1-4614-1527-5 (eBook)
DOI 10.1007/978-1-4614-1527-5
Springer New York Heidelberg Dordrecht London

Library of Congress Control Number: 2011942260

Printed on acid-free paper

Springer is part of Springer Science+Business Media (www.springer.com)

To my parents Mükerrem and Nihat Kitapçı
with deepest gratitude…

MTK

Preface

Integrated positron emission tomography (PET) with computed tomography (CT) has been increasingly used in cancer diagnosis and management. This new imaging tool combines two scan techniques in one exam merging those two (PET and CT) into one set of images combining the usefulness and reducing the limitations of those two distinct imaging modalities.

This book grew out of discussions among the radiologists and nuclear medicine specialists about the limitations of PET and CT. It is an important fact that functional changes in tumor processes happen before morphological changes. Therefore, PET has been a valuable tool in oncology. It is well known that attenuation, which is the loss of detection of true coincidence events, remains as an important challenge when PET images are used alone. This makes harder to interpret particularly in cancer diagnostic and staging images or radiotherapy treatment planning. Meanwhile, CT, providing detailed cross-sectional views of all tissues, is one of the best and fastest tools in morphological imaging. Using those two techniques has grown particular interest in recent years. For PET/CT, CT-scan parameters need to be optimized to minimize radiation exposure to the patient. This optimization requires not giving contrast agents and having less quality images than regular conventional diagnostic CT images taken with the higher scan parameters and with longer time of radiation exposure. We believe it is essential to reeducate ourselves for better evaluation of those lower quality images which are normally used for PET/CT hybrid imaging.

We certainly hope that this atlas will be a user friendly guide to nuclear physicians, radiologists, clinicians, and medical students to consider three dimensions in the mind's eye and the interpretation of the PET/CT properly.

I express my deep gratitude to my mentor and dear friend Dr. R. Edward Coleman for encouraging this work. Certainly producing this book needed time, professional work and collaboration. I want to thank my dear friend Nadir Gülekon, MD, for all his great work with the expertise of being an anatomist as well as a clinical radiologist. I thank for those valuable images taken in Integra Imaging Center and my colleagues M. Ali Gürses, MD and Burcu E. Akkaş, MD. I also thank Andrew Moyer, editor of radiology and nuclear medicine at Springer for the valuable efforts and patience in ensuring the successful publication of this book. Finally I thank my lovely wife Ayşın for her remarks and patience.

Ankara Mehmet T. Kitapçı, MD

Contents

Contributors

Burcu Esen Akkaş, M.D. Abdurrahman Yurtaslan Ankara Oncology Education and Research Hospital, Ankara, Turkey

İ. Nadir Gülekon, M.D., Ph.D. Department of Anatomy, Gazi University, School of Medicine, Ankara, Turkey

Mehmet Ali Gürses, M.D. Integra Medical Imaging Center, Ankara, Turkey

Mehmet T. Kitapçı, M.D. Department of Nuclear Medicine, Gazi University, School of Medicine, Consultant at Integra Medical Imaging Center, Ankara, Turkey

Chapter 1
Head and Neck

M.T. Kitapçı, *Atlas of Sectional Radiological Anatomy for PET/CT*,
DOI 10.1007/978-1-4614-1527-5_1, © Springer Science+Business Media New York 2012

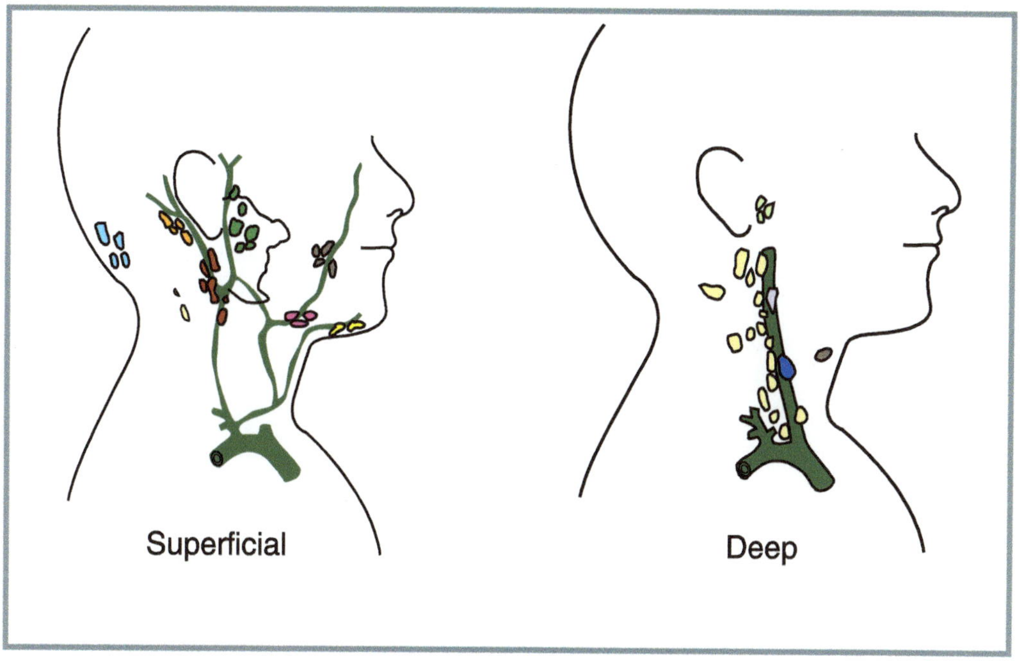

HEAD - NECK

Lymph Nodes

Superficial
Occipital
Retroauricular
Parotid
Buccal
Submental
Submandibular
Superficial cervical

Deep
Jugulo-omohyoid
Deep cervical
Retropharyngeal
Jugulodigastric
Infrahyoid

Adapted and modified from Moore KL, et al.

* *Moore KL, Dalley AF. II. Clinically Oriented Anatomy. 4th ed. Philadelphia: Lippincott Williams & Wilkins, 1999.*

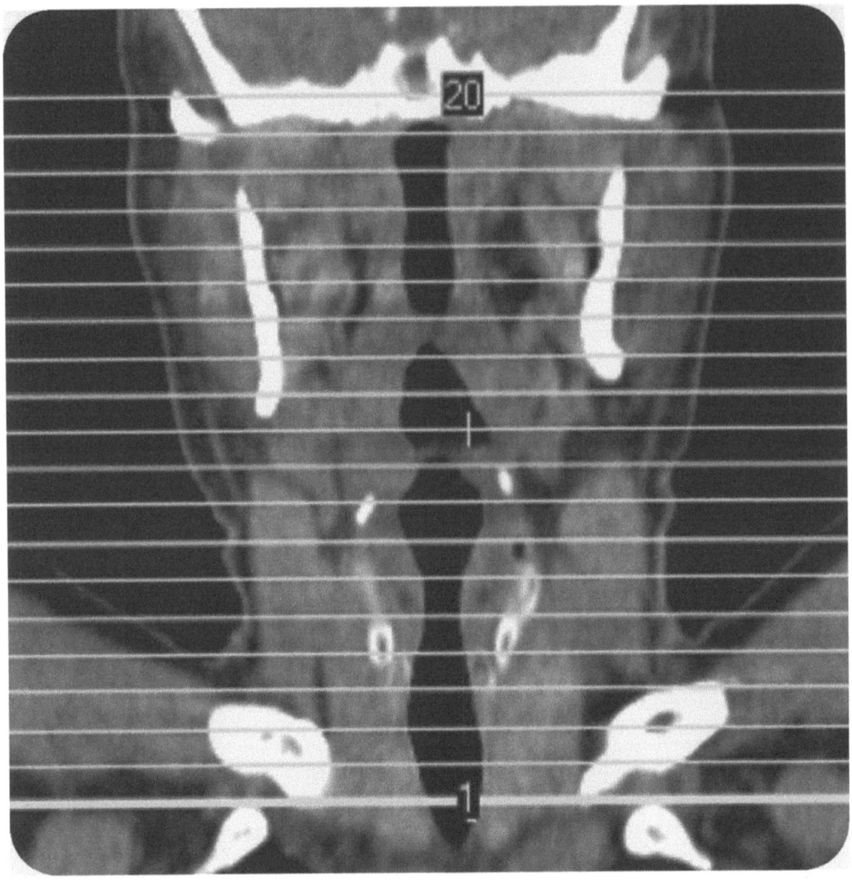

Head and Neck

Consecutive sections were obtained with 3-mm slice thickness and without intravenous contrast. Positron Emission Tomography (PET) and Computed Tomography (CT) images obtained from the same level were given side to side for comparison. All anatomic structures in an image were numbered and given in the explanation section at the bottom of the page. Vertebral levels were marked on each vertebra.

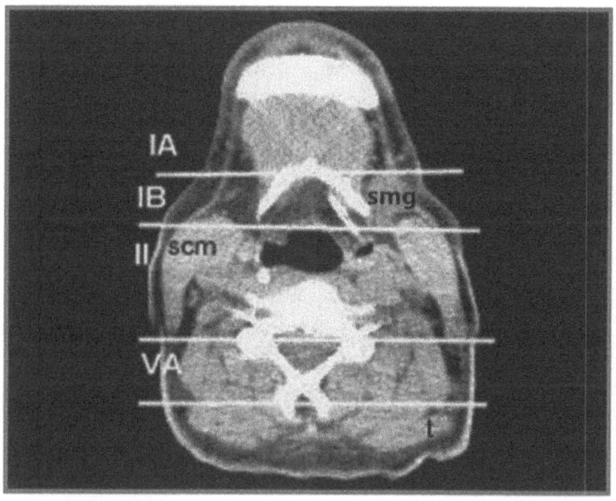

Fig. 1.1 Axial scan at the level of the hyoid bone (*scm* sternocleidomastoid muscle, *smg* submandibular gland, *t* trapezius muscle)

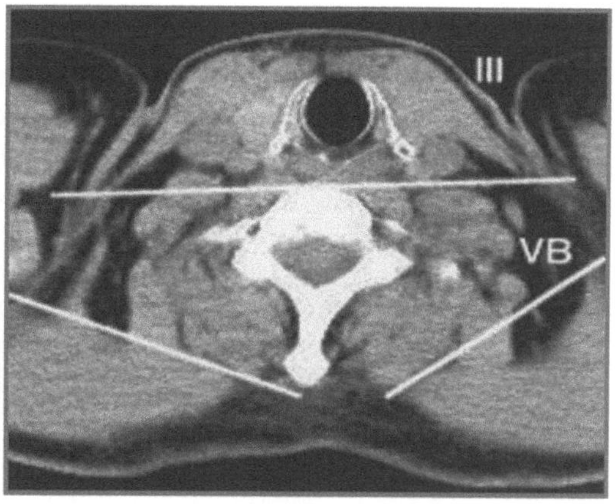

Fig. 1.2 Axial scan at the level of the bottom of the cricoid arch

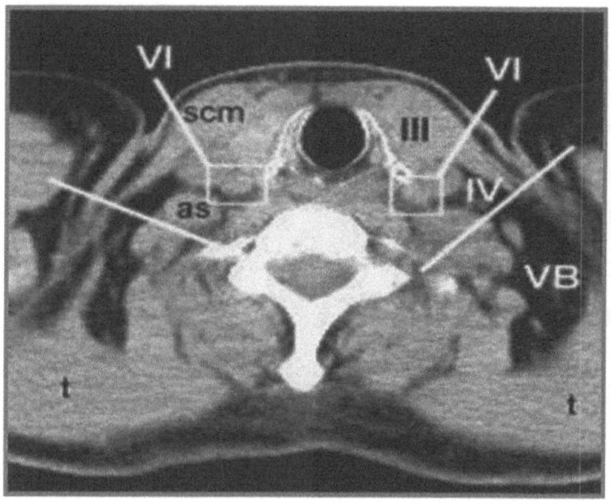

Fig. 1.3 Axial scan at the level of the bottom of the cricoid arch (*scm* sternocleidomastoid muscle, *as* anterior scalene muscle, *t* trapezius muscle)

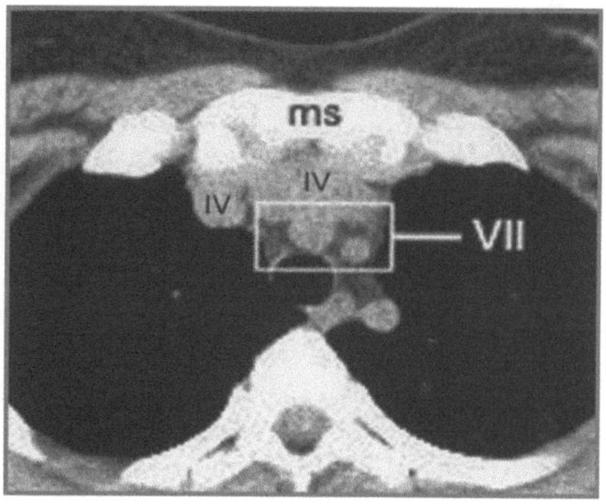

Fig. 1.4 Axial scan at the level of the *upper* mediastinum (*ms* manubrium sterni, *iv* innominate vein)

Keys

Level I The submental and submandibular nodes. They lie above the hyoid bone, below the mylohyoid muscle, and anterior to the back of the submandibular gland (sbg) (Fig. 1.1)

- **Level IA** The submental nodes. They lie between the medial margins of the anterior bellies of the digastric muscle.
- **Level IB** The submandibular nodes. On each side, they lie lateral to the level IA nodes and anterior to the back of each submandibular gland.

Level II The upper internal jugular nodes. They extend from the skull base to the level of the bottom of the body of the hyoid bone. They are posterior to the back of the submandibular gland and anterior to the back of the sternocleidomastoid muscle (scm) (Fig. 1.1).

- **Level IIA** A level II node that lies either anterior, medial, lateral or posterior to the internal jugular vein. If posterior to the vein, the node is inseparable from the vein.
- **Level IIB** A level II node that lies posterior to the internal jugular vein and has a fat plane separating it and the vein.

Level III The middle jugular nodes. They extend from the level of the bottom of the body of the hyoid bone to the level of the bottom of the cricoid arch. They lie anterior to the back of the sternocleidomastoid muscle (Fig. 1.2).

Level IV The low jugular nodes. They extend from the level of the bottom of the cricoid arch to the level of the clavicle. They lie anterior to a line connecting the back of the sternocleidomastoid muscle and the posterolateral margin of the anterior scalene muscle (as). They are also lateral to the carotid arteries (Fig. 1.3).

Level V The nodes in the posterior triangle. They lie posterior to the back of the sternocleidomastoid muscle from the skull base to the level of the bottom of the cricoid arch and posterior to a line connecting the back of the sternocleidomastoid muscle and the posterolateral margin of the anterior scalene muscle from the level of the bottom of the cricoid arch to the level of the clavicle. They also lie anterior to the anterior edge of the trapezius muscle (t) (Figs. 1.1, 1.2, and 1.3).

- **Level VA** Upper level V nodes extend from the skull base to the level of the bottom of the cricoid arch.
- **Level VB** Upper level V nodes extend from the level of the bottom of the cricoid arch to the level of the clavicle, as seen on each axial scan.

Level VI The upper visceral nodes. They lie between the carotid arteries from the level of the bottom of the body of the hyoid bone to the level of the top of the manubrium sterni (ms) (Fig. 1.3).

Level VII The superior mediastinal nodes. They lie between the carotid arteries below the level of the top of the manubrium and above the level of the innominate vein (iv) (Fig. 1.4).

Supraclavicular nodes They lie at or caudal to the level of the clavicle and lateral to the carotid artery on each side of the **nodes** of the neck, as seen on each axial scan.

Retropharyngeal nodes Within 2 cm of the skull base, they lie medial to the internal carotid arteries.

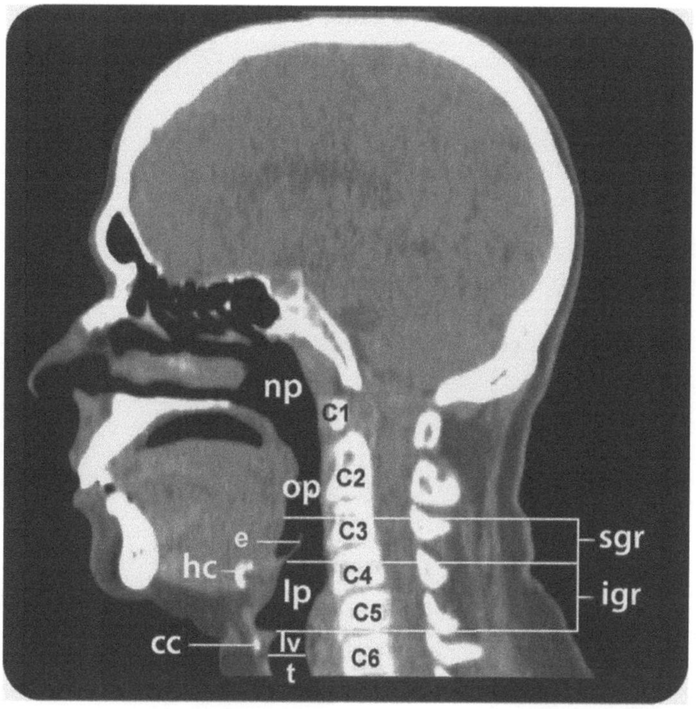

np – nasopharynx
op – oropharynx
e – epiglottis
hc – hyoid cartilage/bone
lp – laryngopharynx
cc – cricoid cartilage
lv – laryngeal vestibule
t – trachea
sgr – supraglottic region
igr – infraglottic region

References

1. Mancuso AA, Harnsberger HR, Muraki AS, Stevens MH. Computed tomography of cervical and retropharyngeal lymph nodes: normal anatomy, variants of normal, and applications in staging head and neck carcinoma, parts I and II. Radiology 1983;148:709–23.
2. Silverman PM. Lymph node imaging: multidetector CT. Cancer Imaging 2005;5:57–67.
3. Som PM, Curtin HO, Mancuso AA. An imaging-based classification for the cervical nodes designed as an adjunct to recent clinically based nodal classifications. Arch Otolaryngol Head Neck Surg 1999;125:388–96.
4. Som PM, Curtin HO, Mancuso AA. Imaging-based nodal classification for evaluation of neck metastatic adenopathy. AJR Am J Roentgenol 2000;174:837–44.

Picture 1

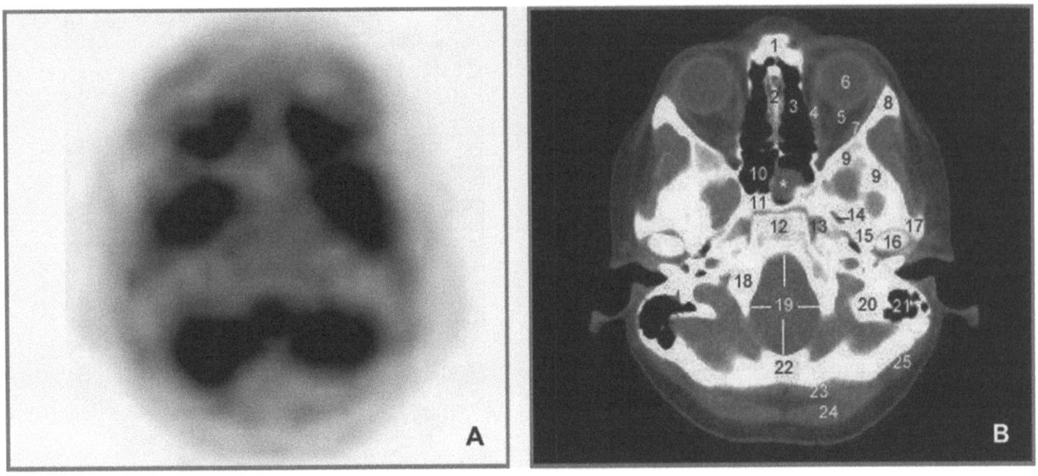

Picture 2

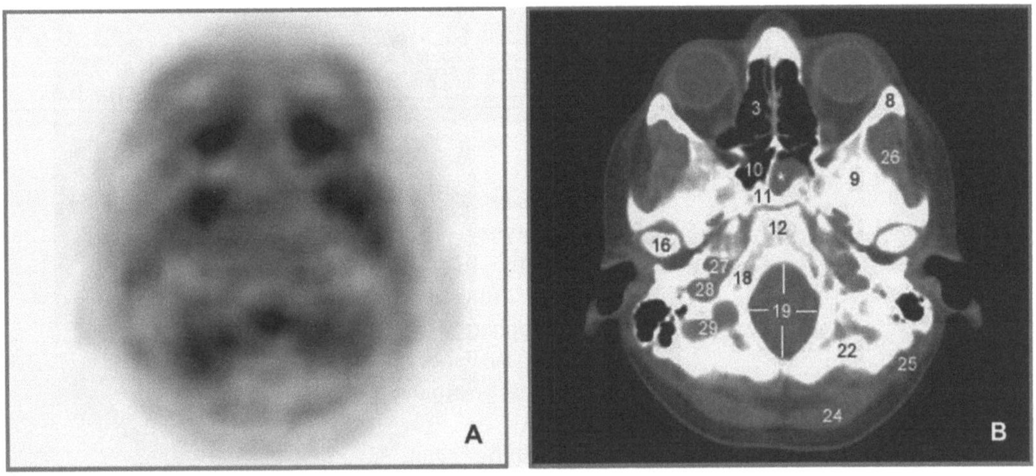

Keys

1. Nasal spine of frontal bone
2. Perpendicular plate of ethmoid bone
3. Ethmoidal air cells
4. Rectus medialis
5. Optic nerve
6. Eyeball
7. Rectus lateralis
8. Frontal process of zygomatic bone
9. Greater wing of sphenoid bone
10. Sphenoidal sinus
11. Body of sphenoid bone
12. Basilar part of occipital bone
13. Foramen lacerum
14. Foramen ovale
15. Petrous part of temporal bone
16. Head of mandible
17. Zygomatic process of temporal bone
18. Lateral part of occipital bone
19. Foramen magnum
20. Mastoid process of temporal bone
21. Mastoid air cells
22. Squamous part of occipital bone
23. Semispinalis capitis
24. Trapezius
25. Splenius capitis
26. Temporalis
27. Internal carotid artery
28. Internal jugular vein
29. Sigmoid sinus

*Mucosal thickening

Picture 3

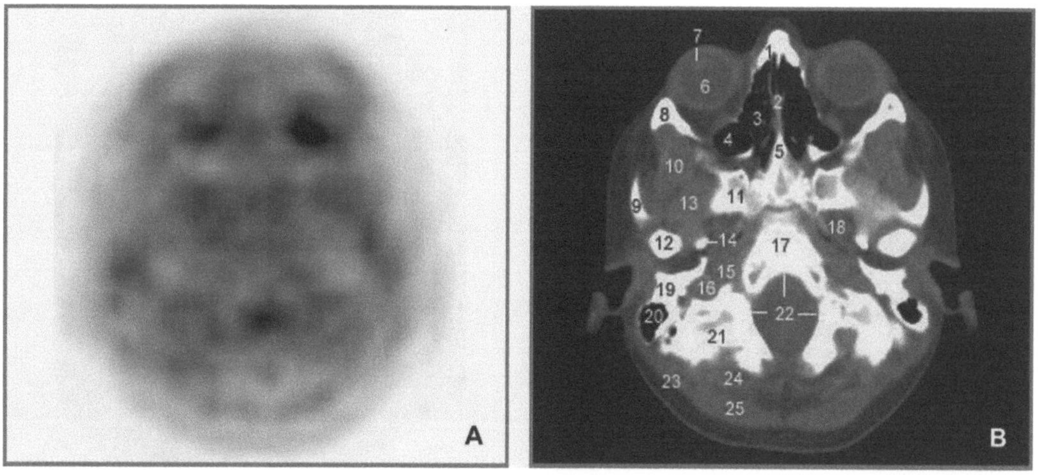

Picture 4

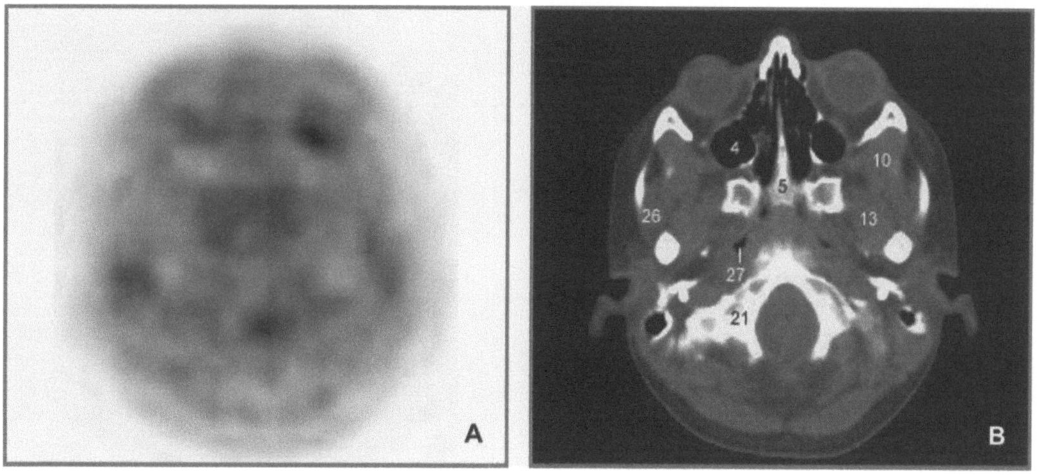

Keys

1. Nasal bone
2. Nasal septum
3. Ethmoidal air cells
4. Maxillary sinus
5. Vomer
6. Eyeball
7. Lens
8. Zygomatic bone
9. Zygomatic arch
10. Temporalis
11. Greater wing of sphenoid bone
12. Head of mandible
13. Lateral pterygoid
14. Styloid process
15. Internal carotid artery
16. Internal jugular vein
17. Basilar part of occipital bone
18. Levator and tensor veli palatini
19. Mastoid process
20. Mastoid air cells
21. Occipital bone
22. Foramen magnum
23. Splenius capitis
24. Semispinalis capitis
25. Trapezius
26. Masseter
27. Auditory tube

Picture 5

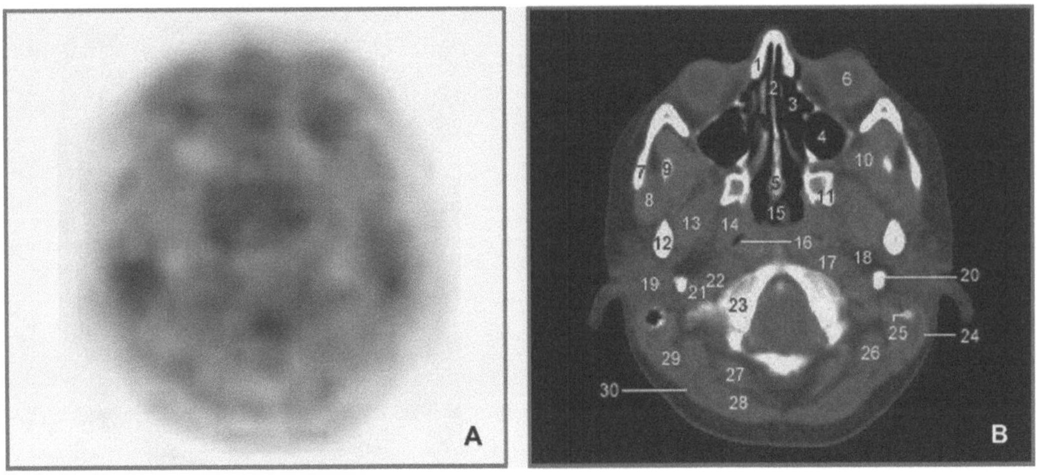

Picture 6

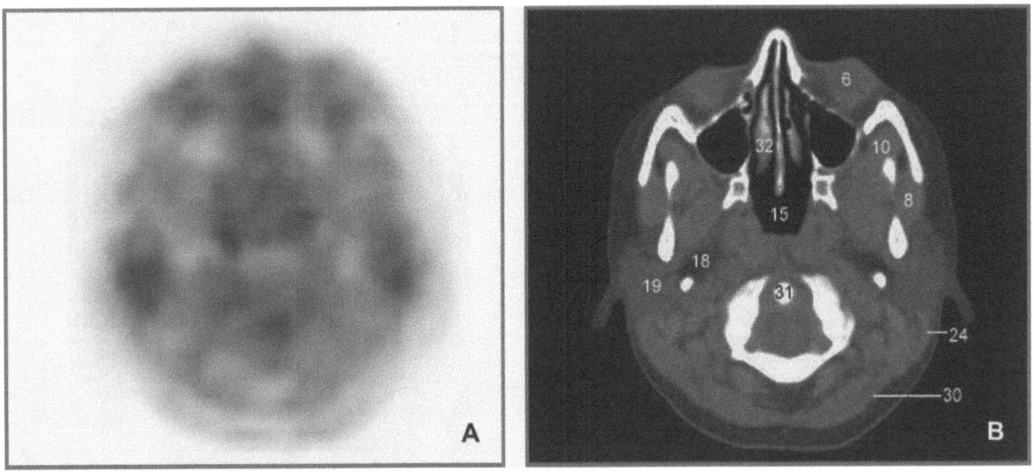

Keys

1. Nasal bone
2. Nasal septum
3. Ethmoidal air cells
4. Maxillary sinus
5. Vomer
6. Eyeball
7. Zygomatic arch
8. Masseter
9. Coronoid process of mandible
10. Temporalis
11. Lateral plate of pterygoid process
12. Neck of mandible
13. Lateral pterygoid muscle
14. Levator and tensor veli palatini
15. Nasopharynx
16. Auditory tube
17. Longus capitis
18. Parapharyngeal space
19. Basilar part of occipital bone
20. Styloid process
21. Internal jugular vein
22. Internal carotid artery
23. Occipital bone
24. Sternocleidomastoid
25. Mastoid process
26. Longissimus capitis
27. Rectus capitis posterior minor
28. Semispinalis capitis
29. Splenius capitis
30. Trapezius
31. Odontoid process of axis (C2)
32. Middle nasal concha

Picture 7

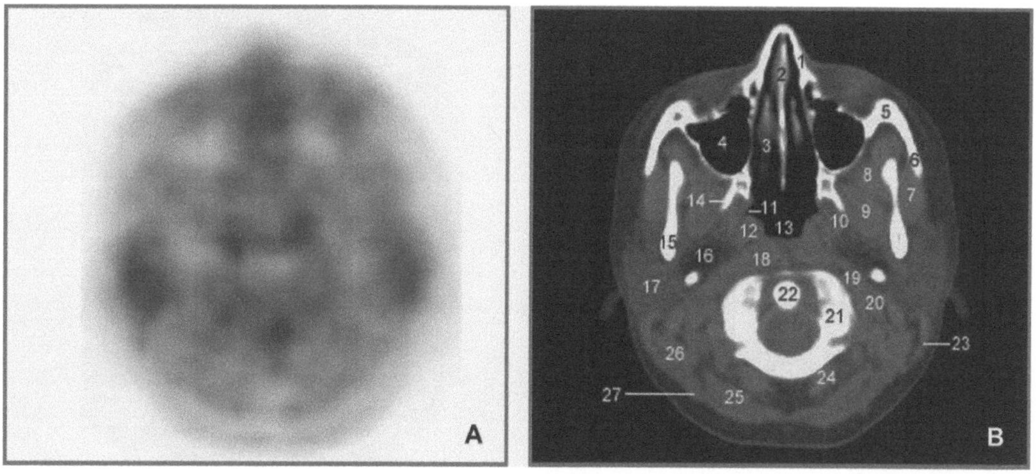

Picture 8

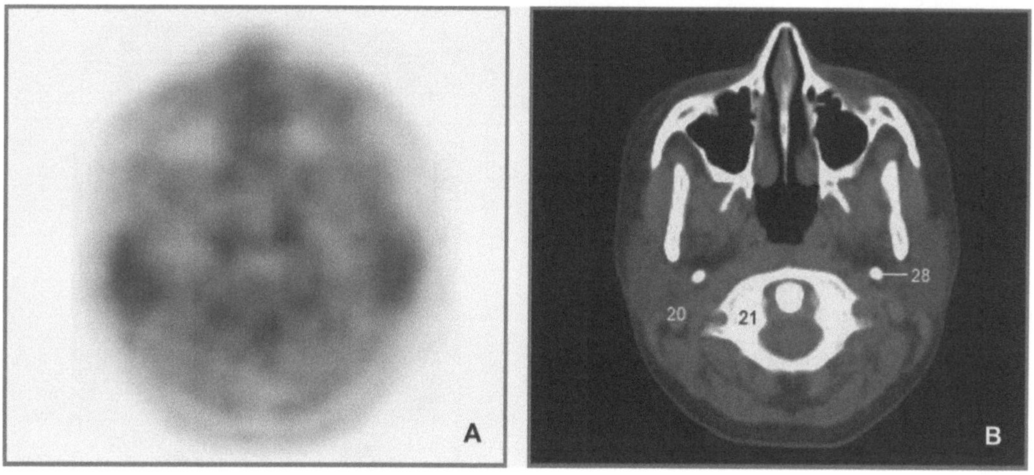

Keys

1. Nasal bone
2. Nasal septum
3. Nasal cavity
4. Maxillary sinus
5. Zygomatic bone
6. Zygomatic arch
7. Masseter
8. Temporalis
9. Lateral pterygoid muscle
10. Tensor veli palatini
11. Nasopharynx
12. Levator veli palatini
13. Pharyngeal recess (Rosenmüller's fossa)
14. Lateral plate of pterygoid process
15. Ramus of mandible
16. Parapharyngeal space
17. Parotid gland
18. Longus capitis
19. Internal carotid artery
20. Internal jugular vein
21. Atlas (C1)
22. Dens axis (C2)
23. Sternocleidomastoid
24. Rectus capitis posterior minor
25. Semispinalis capitis
26. Splenius capitis
27. Trapezius
28. Styloid process

Picture 9

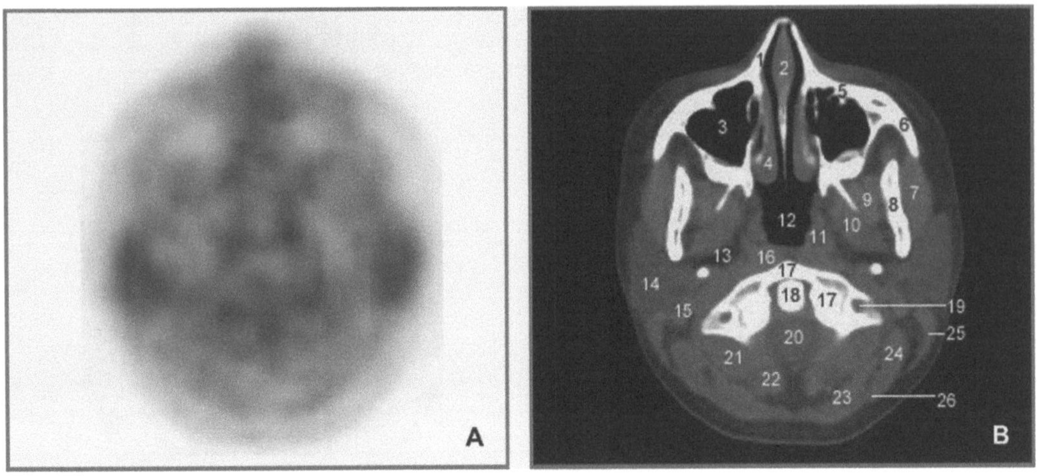

Picture 10

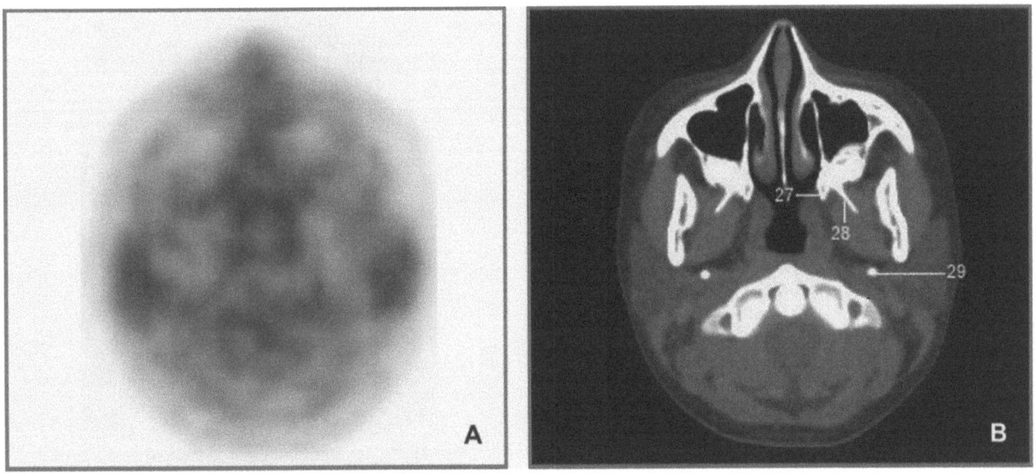

Keys

1. Nasal bone
2. Nasal septum
3. Maxillary sinus
4. Inferior nasal concha
5. Maxilla
6. Zygomatic bone
7. Masseter
8. Ramus of mandible
9. Lateral pterygoid muscle
10. Medial pterygoid muscle
11. Levator and tensor veli palatini
12. Nasopharynx
13. Parapharyngeal space
14. Parotid gland
15. Internal carotid artery and vein
16. Longus capitis
17. Atlas (C1)
18. Dens axis (C2)
19. Foramen transversarium of atlas
20. Spinal cord
21. Obliquus capitis superior
22. Rectus capitis posterior major
23. Semispinalis capitis
24. Splenius capitis
25. Sternocleidomastoid
26. Trapezius
27. Medial plate of pterygoid process
28. Lateral plate of pterygoid process
29. Styloid process

Picture 11

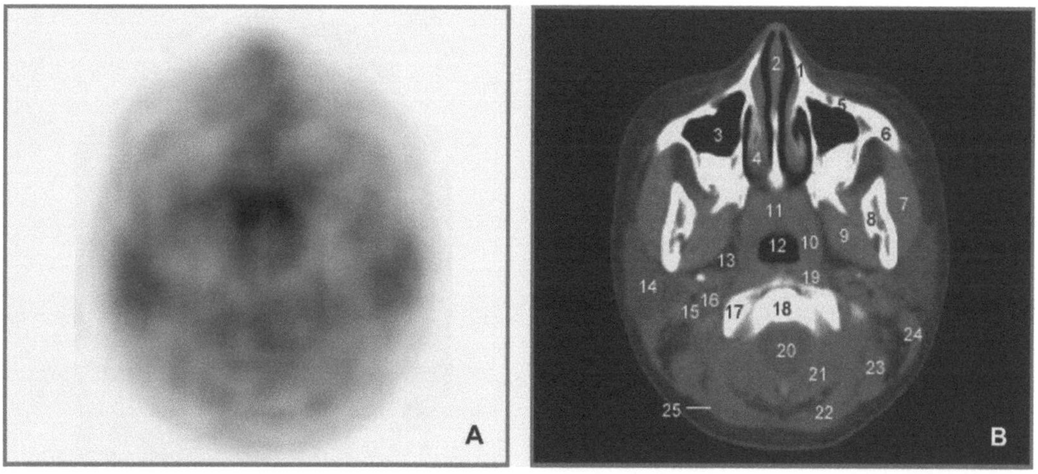

Picture 12

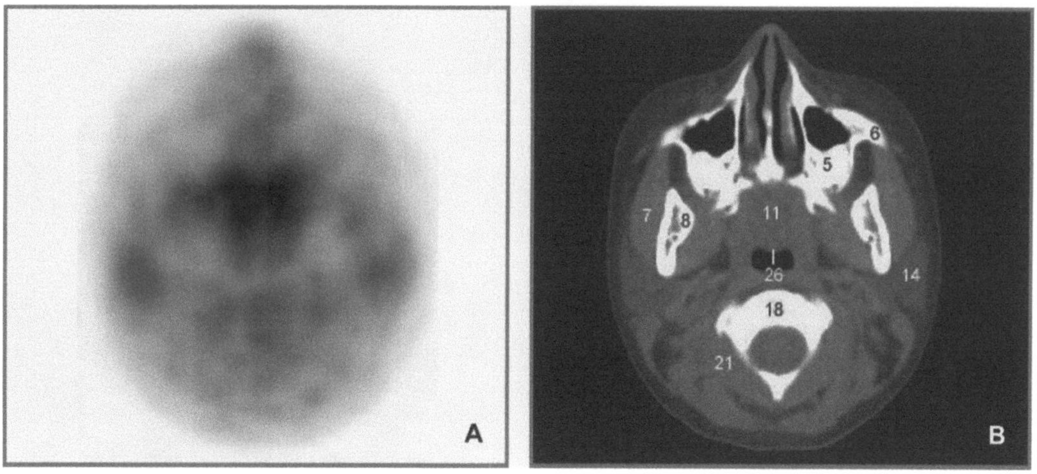

Keys

1. Nasal bone
2. Nasal septum
3. Maxillary sinus
4. Inferior nasal concha
5. Maxilla
6. Zygomatic bone
7. Masseter
8. Ramus of mandible
9. Medial pterygoid muscle
10. Superior pharyngeal constrictor
11. Soft palate
12. Oropharynx
13. Parapharyngeal space
14. Parotid gland
15. Internal jugular vein
16. Internal carotid artery
17. Atlas (C1)
18. Axis (C2)
19. Longus capitis
20. Spinal cord
21. Deep muscles of neck
22. Semispinalis capitis
23. Splenius capitis
24. Sternocleidomastoid
25. Trapezius
26. Uvula

Picture 13

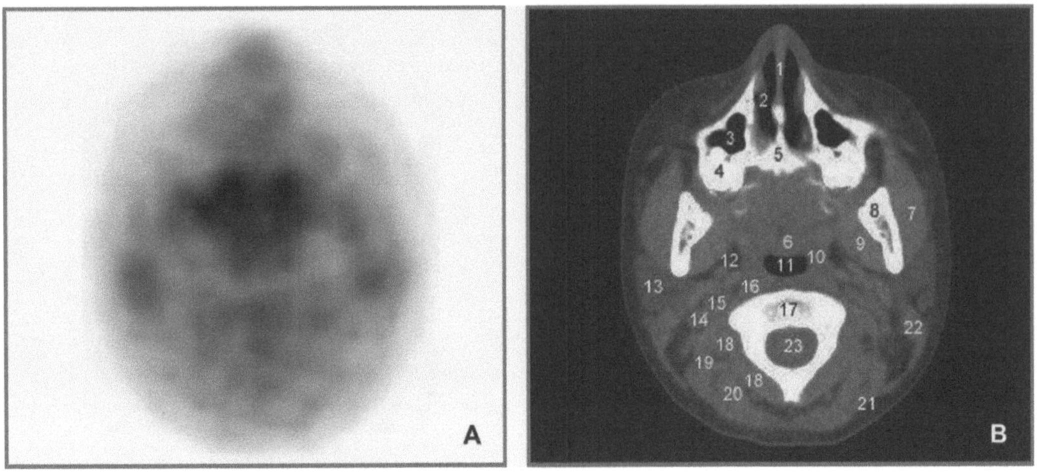

Picture 14

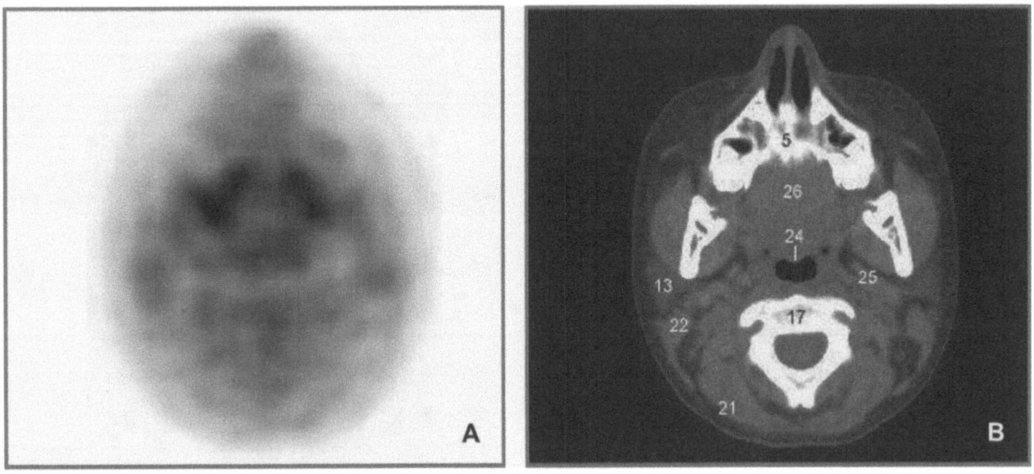

Keys

1. Nasal septum
2. Nasal cavity
3. Maxillary sinus
4. Maxilla
5. Palatine bone
6. Soft palate
7. Masseter
8. Ramus of mandible
9. Medial pterygoid muscle
10. Superior pharyngeal constrictor
11. Oropharynx
12. Parapharyngeal space
13. Parotid gland
14. Internal jugular vein
15. Internal carotid artery
16. Longus capitis
17. Axis (C2)
18. Deep muscles of neck
19. Splenius capitis
20. Semispinalis capitis
21. Trapezius
22. Sternocleidomastoid
23. Spinal cord
24. Uvula
25. External carotid artery
26. Tongue

Picture 15

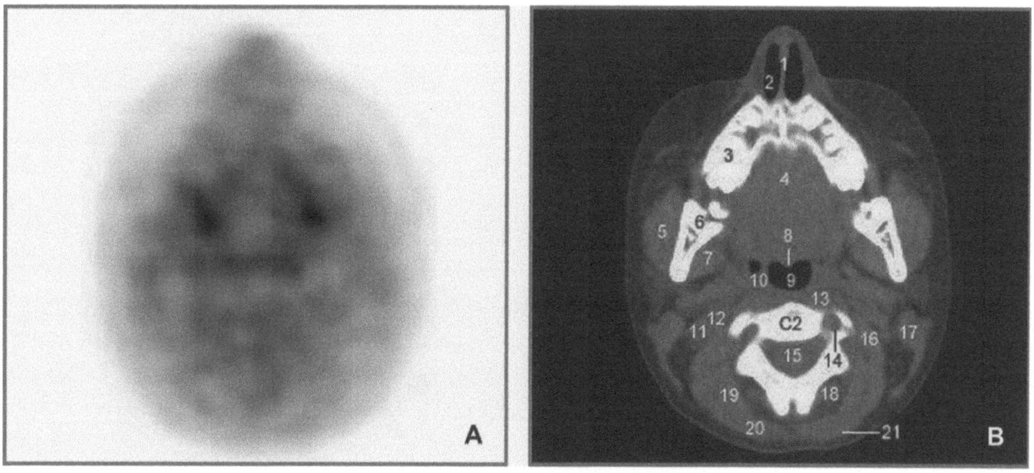

Picture 16

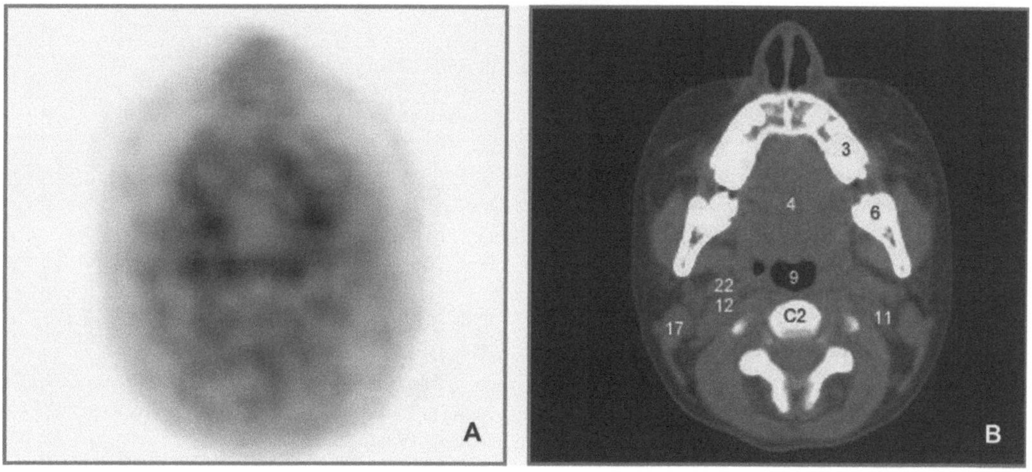

Keys

1. Nasal septum
2. Nasal cavity
3. Alveolar process of maxilla
4. Tongue
5. Masseter
6. Mandible
7. Medial pterygoid muscle
8. Uvula
9. Oropharynx
10. Superior and middle pharyngeal constrictor
11. Internal jugular vein
12. Internal carotid artery
13. Longus capitis and longus colli
14. Foramen transversarium of axis
15. Spinal cord
16. Levator scapulae
17. Sternocleidomastoid
18. Deep muscles of neck
19. Splenius capitis
20. Semispinalis capitis
21. Trapezius
22. External carotid artery

Picture 17

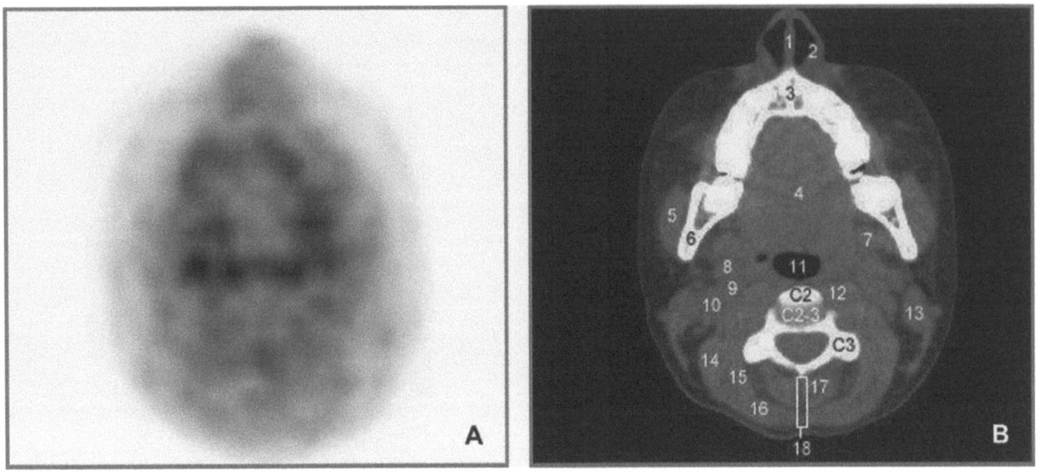

Picture 18

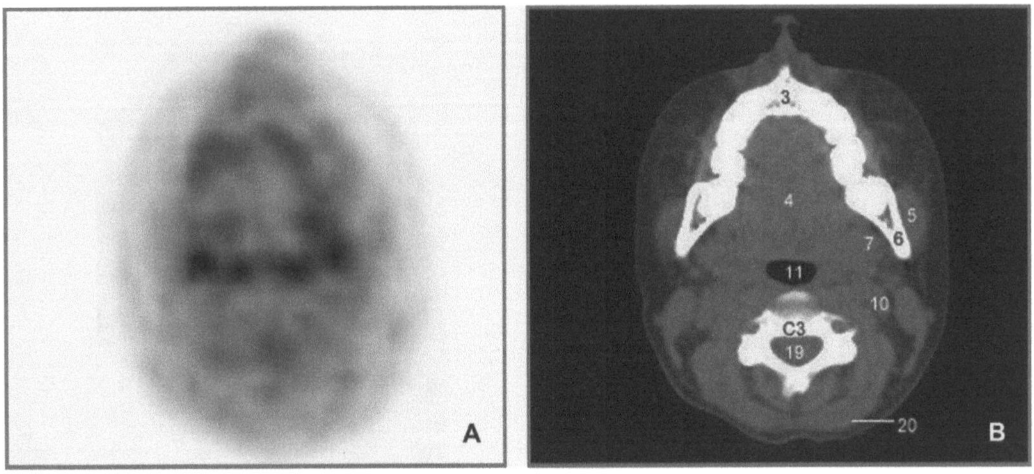

Keys

1. Nasal septum
2. Ala of nose
3. Alveolar process of maxilla
4. Tongue
5. Masseter
6. Mandible
7. Submandibular gland
8. External carotid artery
9. Internal carotid artery
10. Internal jugular vein
11. Oropharynx
12. Longus capitis and longus colli
13. Sternocleidomastoid
14. Levator scapulae
15. Splenius capitis
16. Semispinalis capitis
17. Semispinalis cervicis
18. Nuchal ligament
19. Spinal cord
20. Trapezius

Picture 19

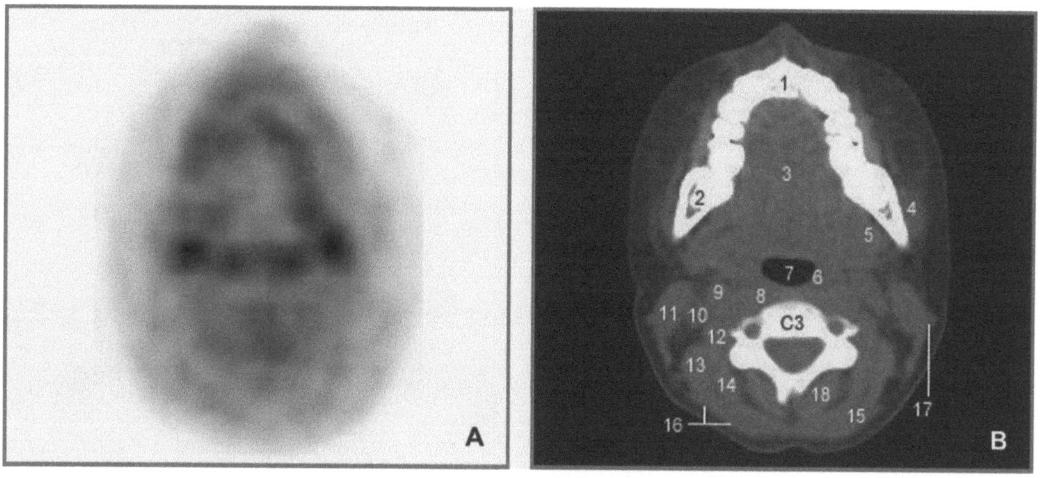

Picture 20

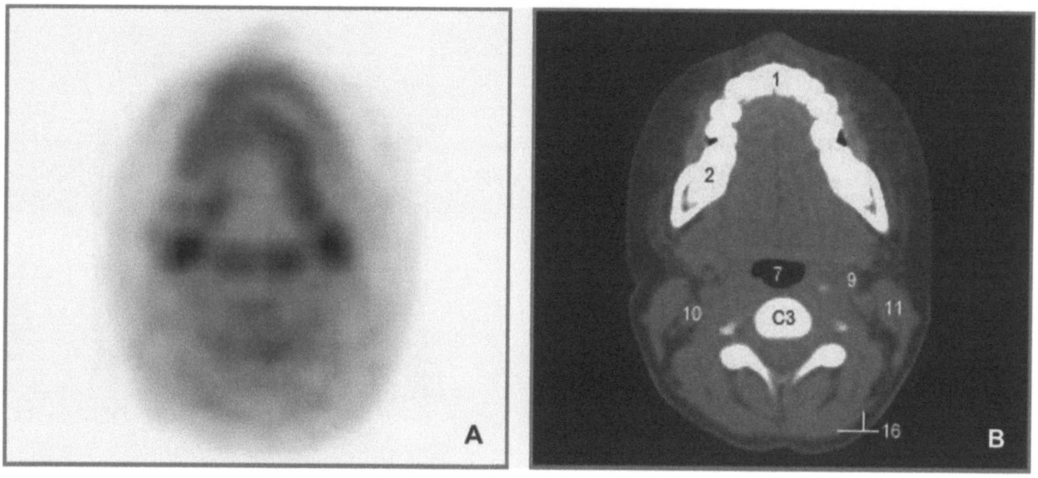

Keys

1. Alveolar process of maxilla
2. Mandible
3. Tongue
4. Masseter
5. Submandibular gland
6. Middle pharyngeal constrictor
7. Oropharynx
8. Longus capitis and longus colli
9. Common carotid artery
10. Internal jugular vein
11. Sternocleidomastoid
12. Longissimus cervicis
13. Levator scapulae
14. Splenius capitis
15. Semispinalis capitis
16. Trapezius
17. External jugular vein
18. Semispinalis cervicis

Picture 21

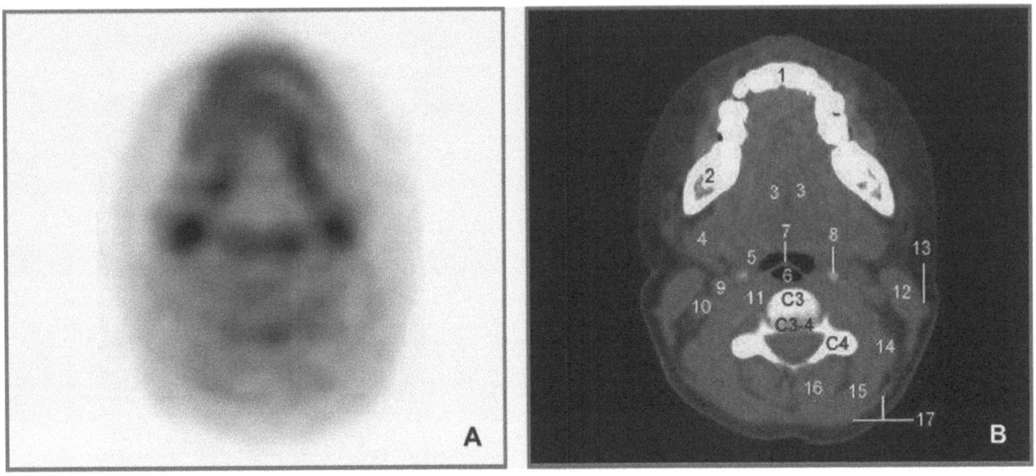

Picture 22

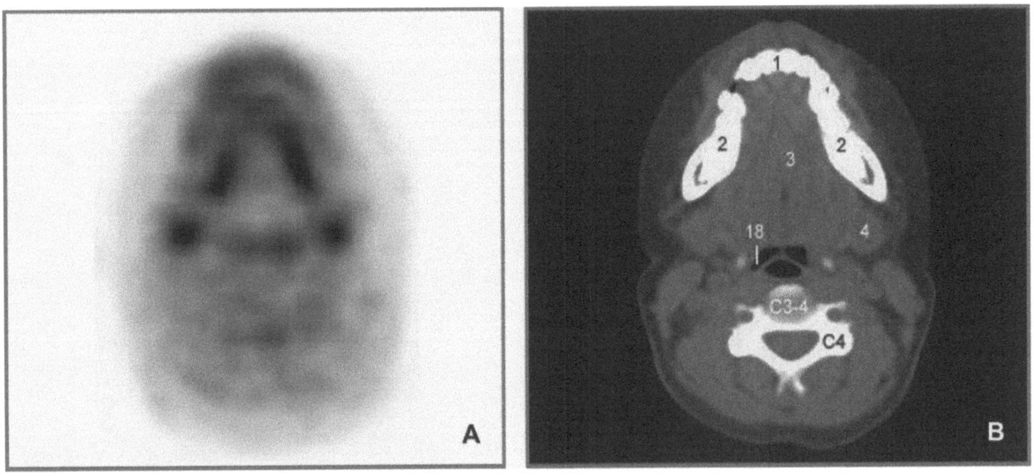

Keys

1. Upper teeth
2. Mandible
3. Genioglossus
4. Submandibular gland
5. Palatine tonsil
6. Laryngopharynx
7. Epiglottic cartilage
8. Hyoid bone
9. Common carotid artery
10. Internal jugular vein
11. Longus capitis and longus colli
12. Sternocleidomastoid
13. External jugular vein
14. Levator scapulae
15. Semispinalis capitis and splenius capitis
16. Semispinalis cervicis
17. Trapezius
18. Piriform fossa

Picture 23

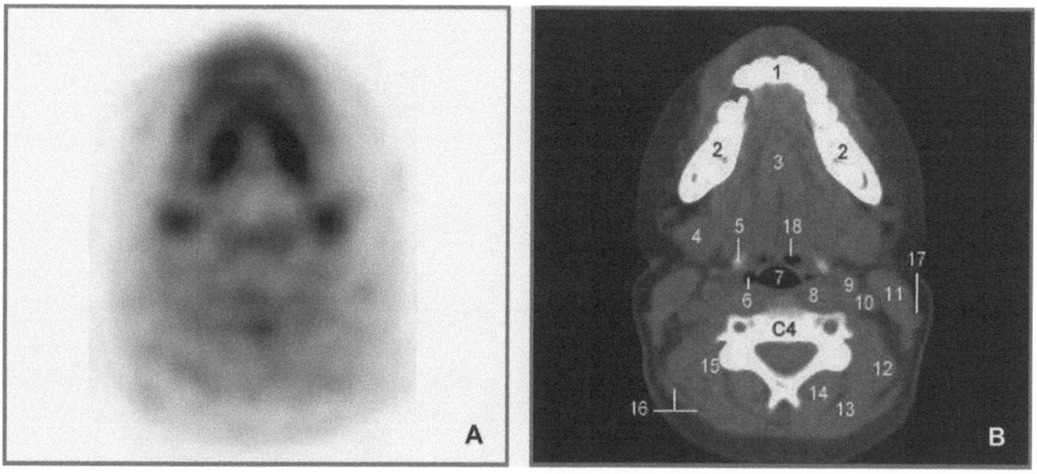

Picture 24

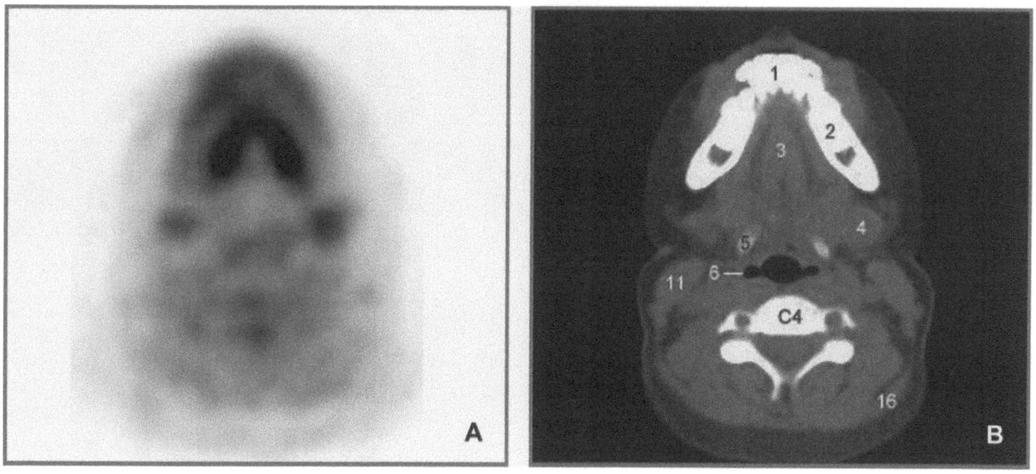

Keys

1. Upper teeth	10. Internal jugular vein
2. Mandible	11. Sternocleidomastoid
3. Geniohyoid	12. Levator scapulae
4. Submandibular gland	13. Semispinalis capitis and splenius capitis
5. Hyoid bone	14. Deep muscles of neck
6. Piriform fossa	15. Longissimus cervicis
7. Laryngopharynx	16. Trapezius
8. Longus capitis and longus colli	17. External jugular vein
9. Common carotid artery	18. Vallecula

Picture 25

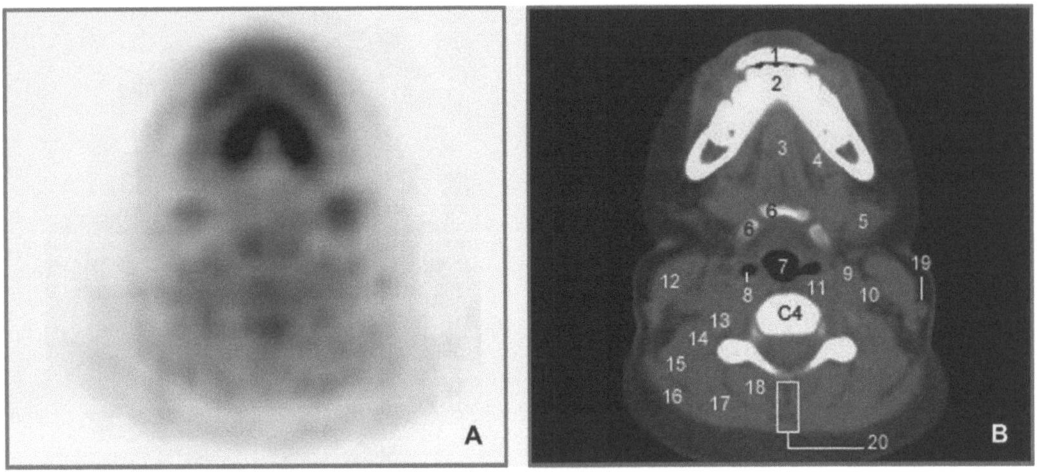

Picture 26

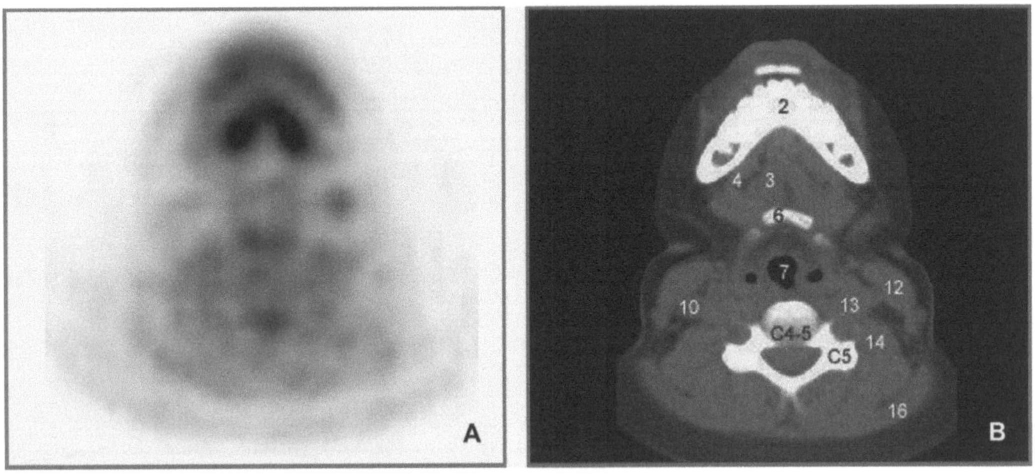

Keys

1. Upper teeth
2. Lower teeth
3. Mylohyoid
4. Anterior belly of digastricus
5. Submandibular gland
6. Hyoid bone
7. Laryngopharynx
8. Piriform fossa
9. Common carotid artery
10. Internal jugular vein
11. Longus capitis and longus colli
12. Sternocleidomastoid
13. Anterior scalene
14. Middle and posterior scalene
15. Levator scapulae
16. Trapezius
17. Semispinalis capitis and splenius capitis
18. Deep muscles of neck
19. External jugular vein
20. Nuchal ligament

Picture 27

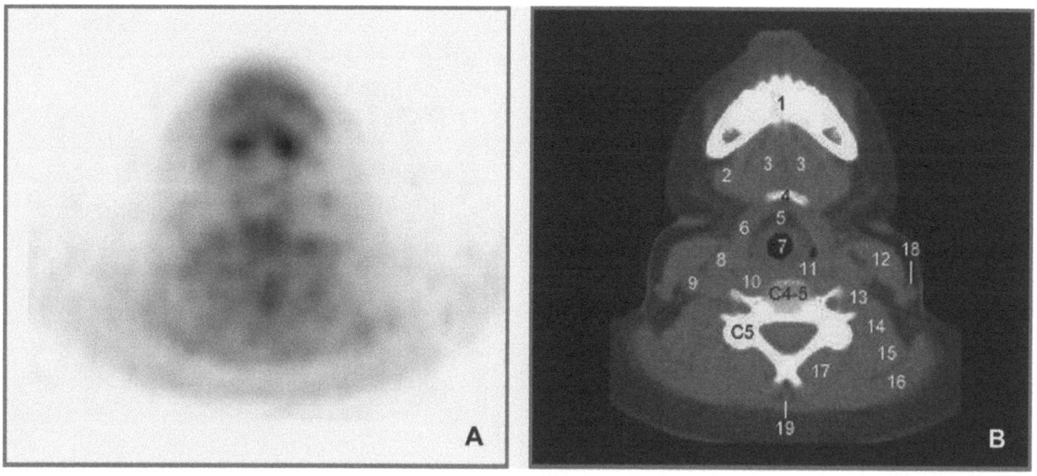

Picture 28

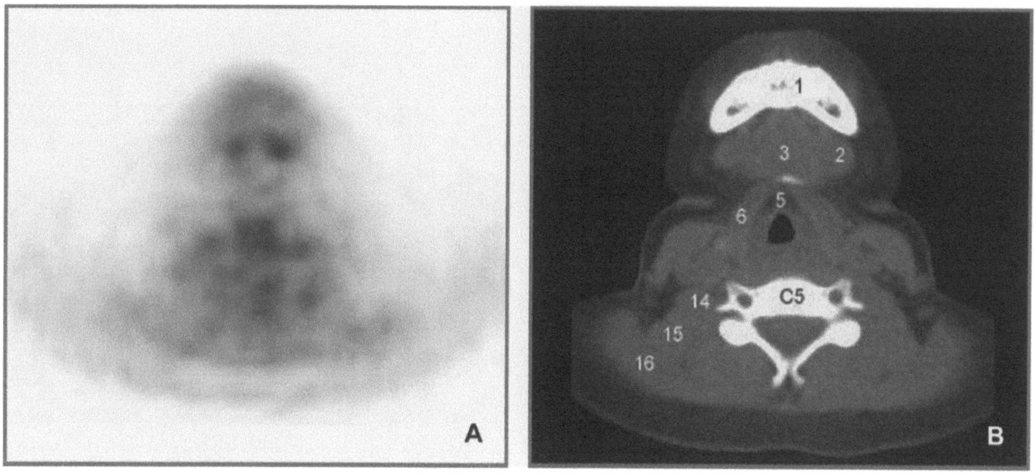

Keys

1. Mandible
2. Anterior belly of digastricus
3. Mylohyoid
4. Hyoid bone
5. Prelaryngeal fat body
6. Infrahyoid muscles
7. Laryngeal vestibule
8. Common carotid artery
9. Internal jugular vein
10. Longus capitis and longus colli
11. Inferior pharyngeal constrictor
12. Sternocleidomastoid
13. Anterior scalene
14. Middle and posterior scalene
15. Levator scapulae
16. Trapezius
17. Deep muscles of neck
18. External jugular vein
19. Nuchal ligament

Picture 29

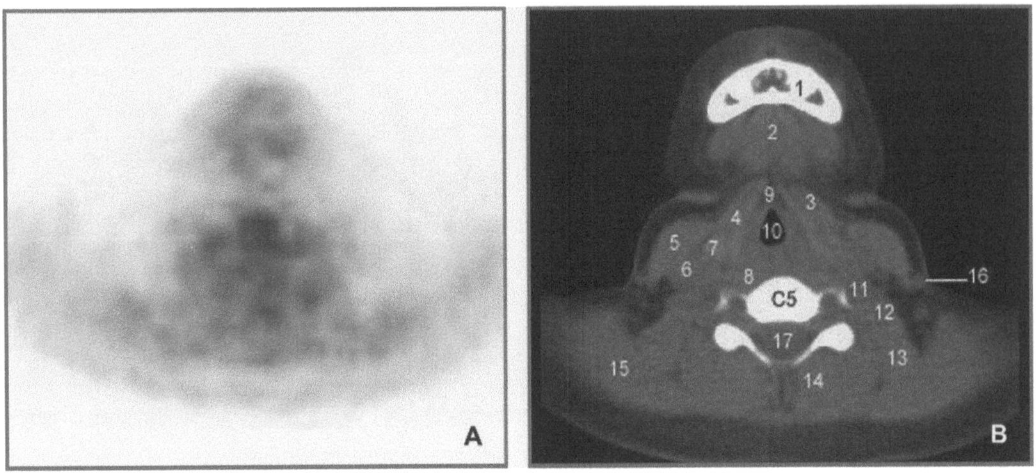

Picture 30

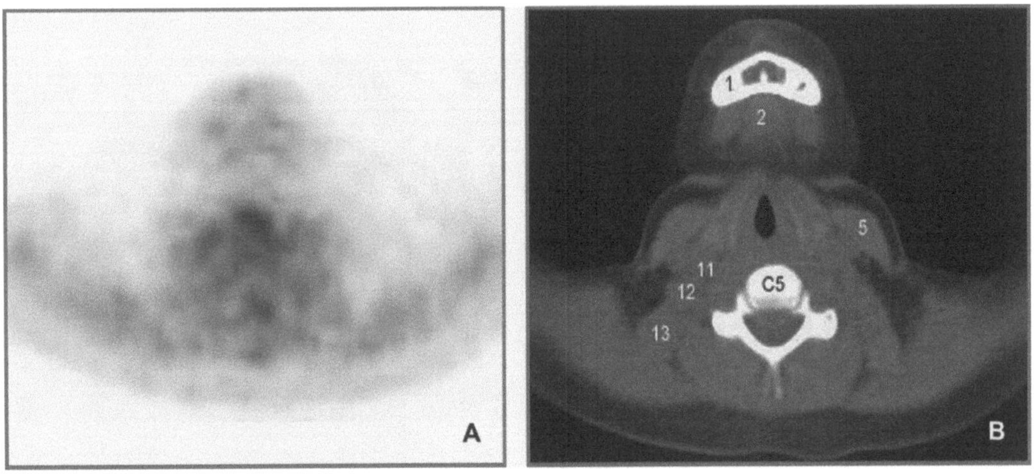

Keys

1. Mandible
2. Mylohyoid
3. Infrahyoid muscles
4. Thyroid cartilage
5. Sternocleidomastoid
6. Internal jugular vein
7. Common carotid artery
8. Longus colli
9. Prelaryngeal fat body
10. Laryngeal vestibule
11. Anterior scalene
12. Middle and posterior scalene
13. Levator scapulae
14. Deep muscles of neck
15. Trapezius
16. External jugular vein
17. Spinal cord

Picture 31

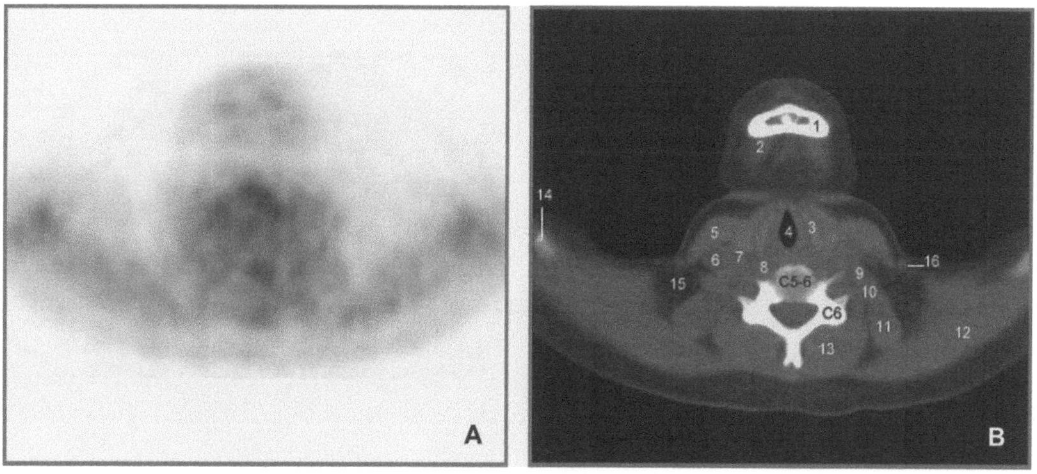

Picture 32

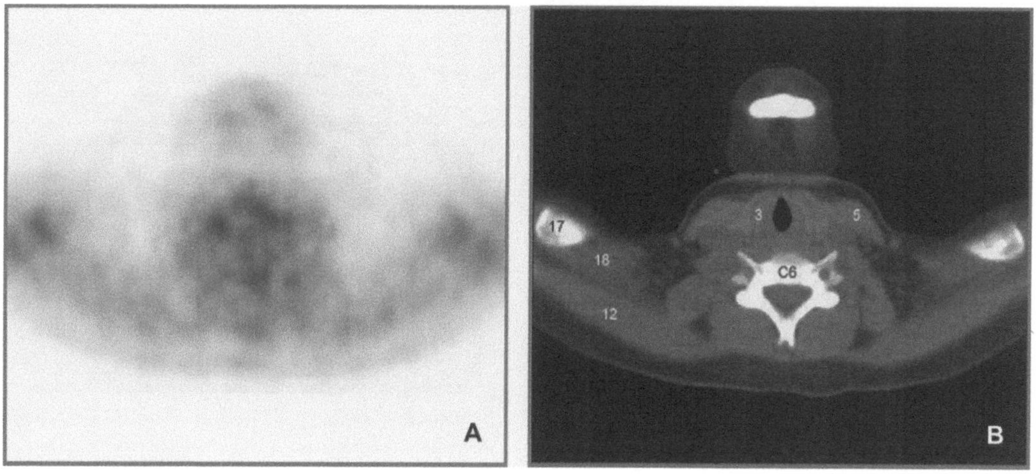

Keys

1. Mandible
2. Mylohyoid
3. Thyroid cartilage
4. Infraglottic cavity
5. Sternocleidomastoid
6. Internal jugular vein
7. Common carotid artery
8. Longus colli
9. Anterior scalene
10. Middle and posterior scalene
11. Levator scapulae
12. Trapezius
13. Deep muscles of neck
14. Acromion
15. Lateral cervical region
16. External jugular vein
17. Acromial end of clavicle
18. Deltoid

Picture 33

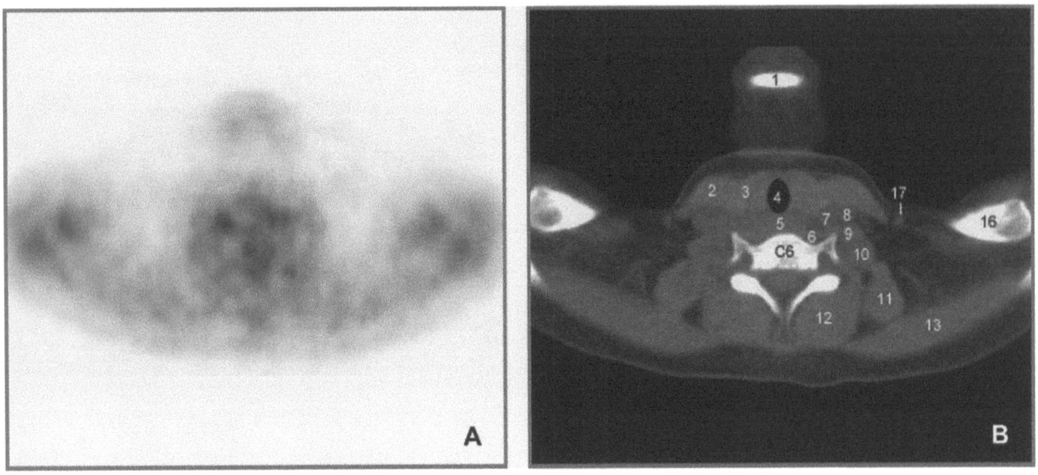

Picture 34

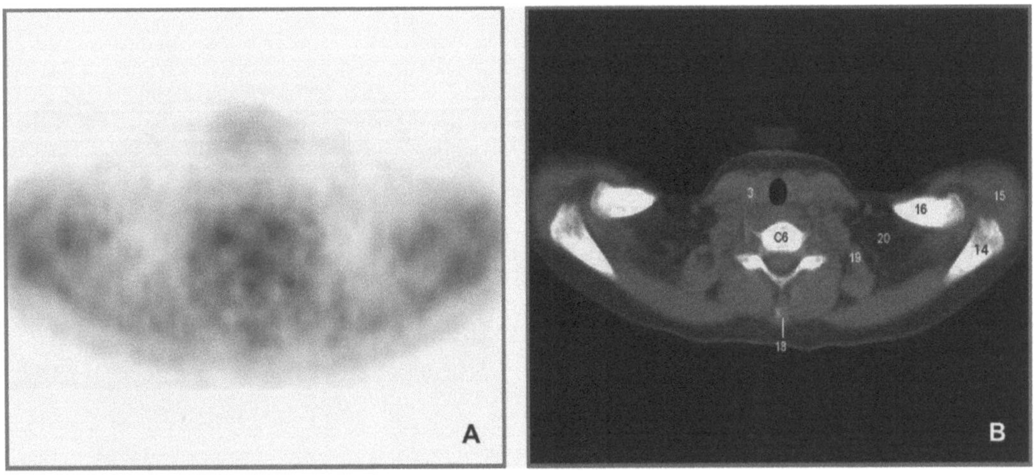

Keys

1. Mandible
2. Sternocleidomastoid
3. Thyroid gland
4. Infraglottic cavity
5. Oesophagus
6. Longus colli
7. Common carotid artery
8. Internal jugular vein
9. Anterior scalene
10. Middle scalene
11. Levator scapulae
12. Deep muscles of neck
13. Trapezius
14. Acromion
15. Deltoid
16. Clavicle
17. External jugular vein
18. Nuchal ligament
19. Posterior scalene
20. Supraclavicular fossa

Picture 35

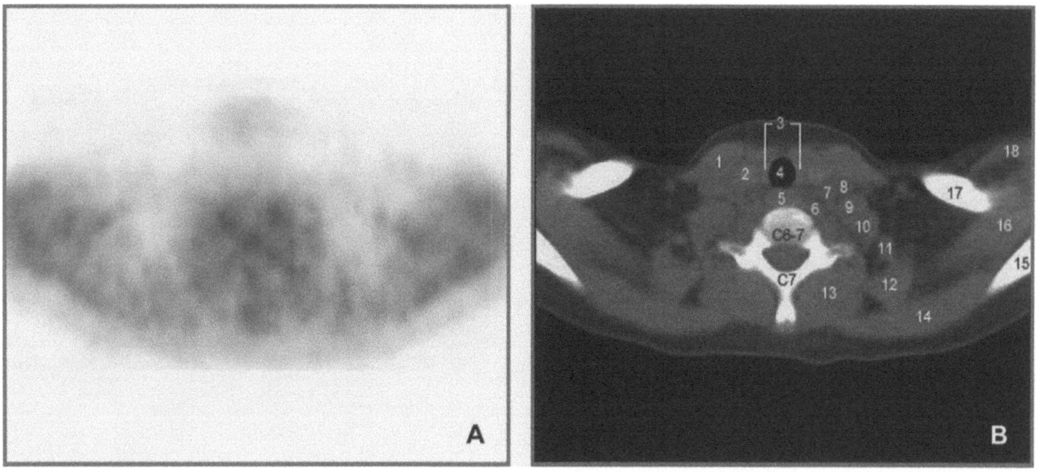

Picture 36

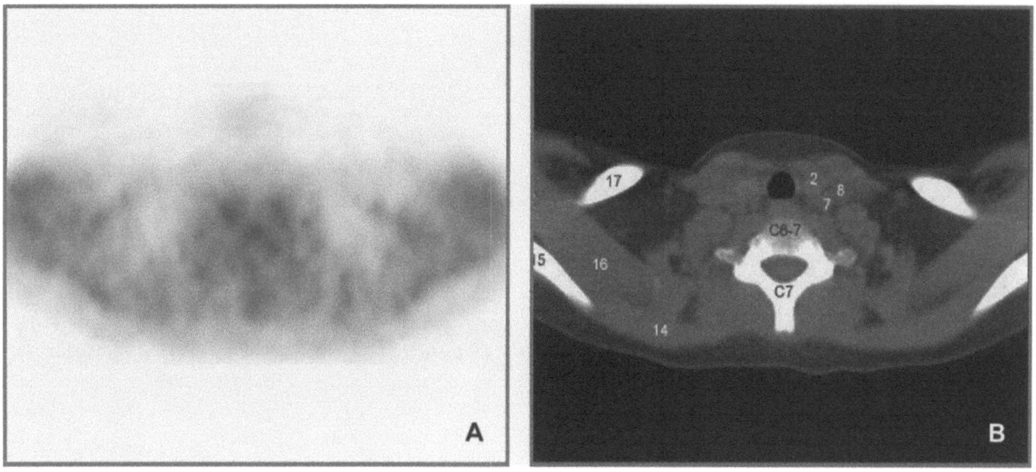

Keys

1. Sternocleidomastoid
2. Thyroid gland
3. Cricoid cartilage
4. Trachea
5. Oesophagus
6. Longus colli
7. Common carotid artery
8. Internal jugular vein
9. Anterior scalene
10. Middle scalene
11. Posterior scalene
12. Levator scapulae
13. Deep muscles of neck
14. Trapezius
15. Scapula
16. Supraspinatus
17. Clavicle
18. Deltoid

Picture 37

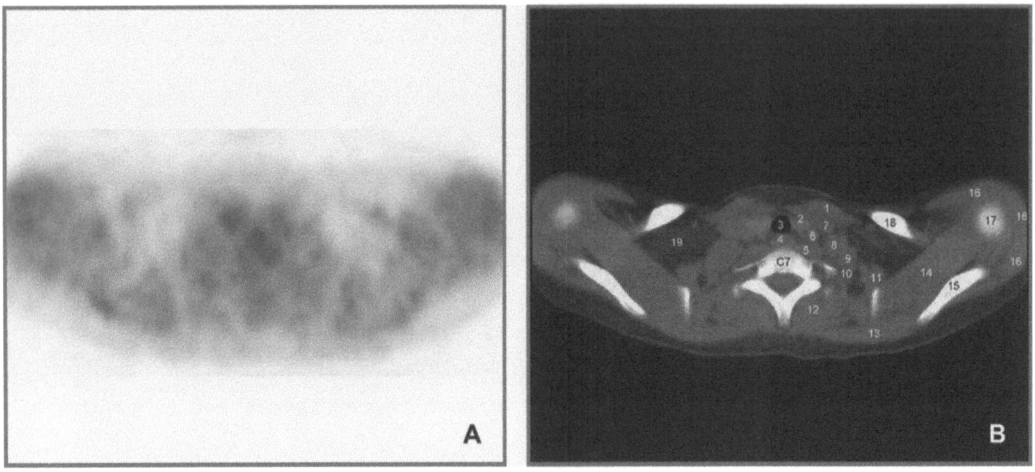

Picture 38

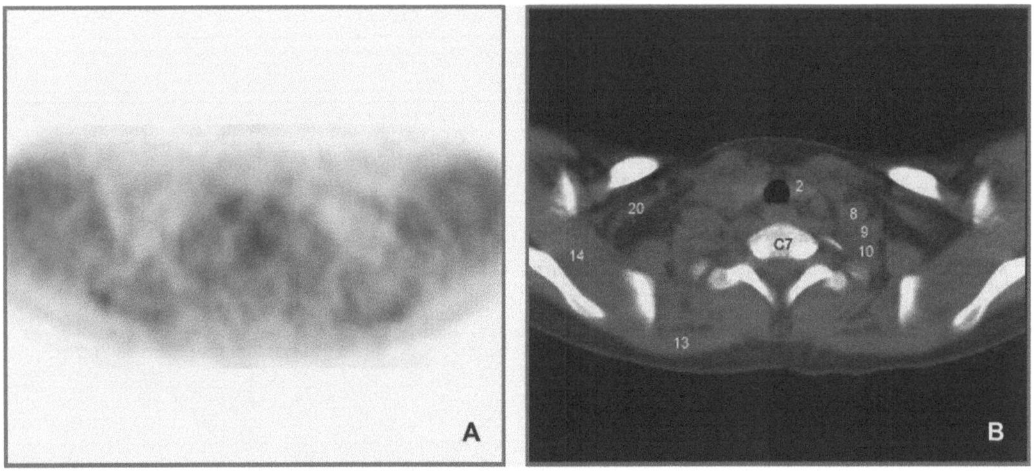

Keys

1. Sternocleidomastoid
2. Thyroid gland
3. Trachea
4. Oesophagus
5. Longus colli
6. Common carotid artery
7. Internal jugular vein
8. Anterior scalene
9. Middle scalene
10. Posterior scalene
11. Levator scapulae
12. Deep muscles of neck
13. Trapezius
14. Supraspinatus
15. Scapula
16. Deltoid
17. Head of humerus
18. Clavicle
19. Supraclavicular fossa
20. Subclavian artery

Picture 39

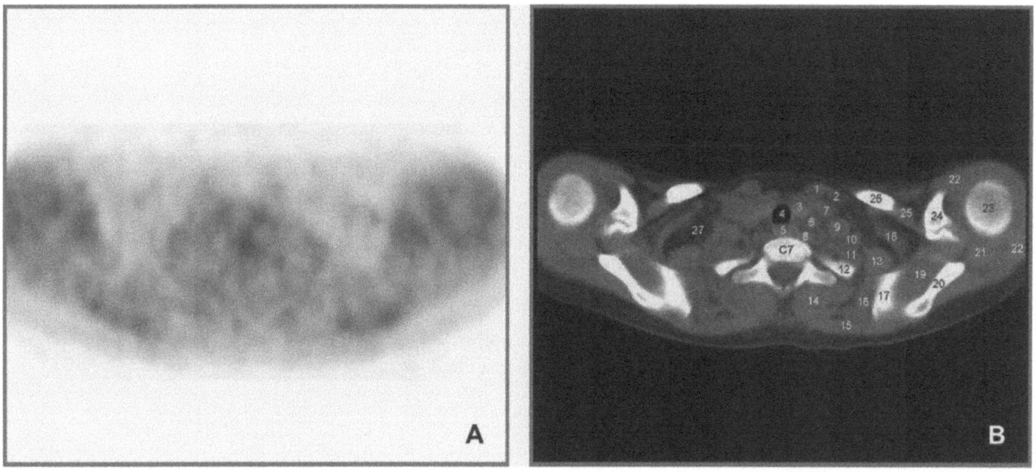

Picture 40

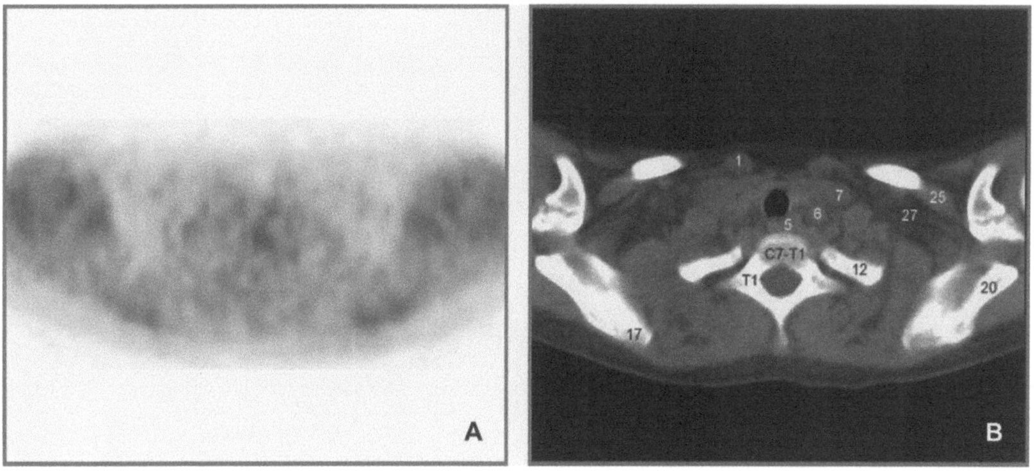

Keys

1. Sternocleidomastoid, sternal head
2. Sternocleidomastoid, clavicular head
3. Thyroid gland
4. Trachea
5. Oesophagus
6. Common carotid artery
7. Internal jugular vein
8. Longus colli
9. Anterior scalene
10. Middle scalene
11. Posterior scalene
12. 1st rib
13. Levator scapulae
14. Deep muscles of neck
15. Trapezius
16. Subscapularis
17. Scapula
18. Subclavian artery
19. Supraspinatus
20. Spine of scapula
21. Infraspinatus
22. Deltoid
23. Head of humerus
24. Neck of scapula
25. Subclavius
26. Clavicle
27. Supraclavicular fossa

Chapter 2
Thorax

M.T. Kitapçı, *Atlas of Sectional Radiological Anatomy for PET/CT*,
DOI 10.1007/978-1-4614-1527-5_2,

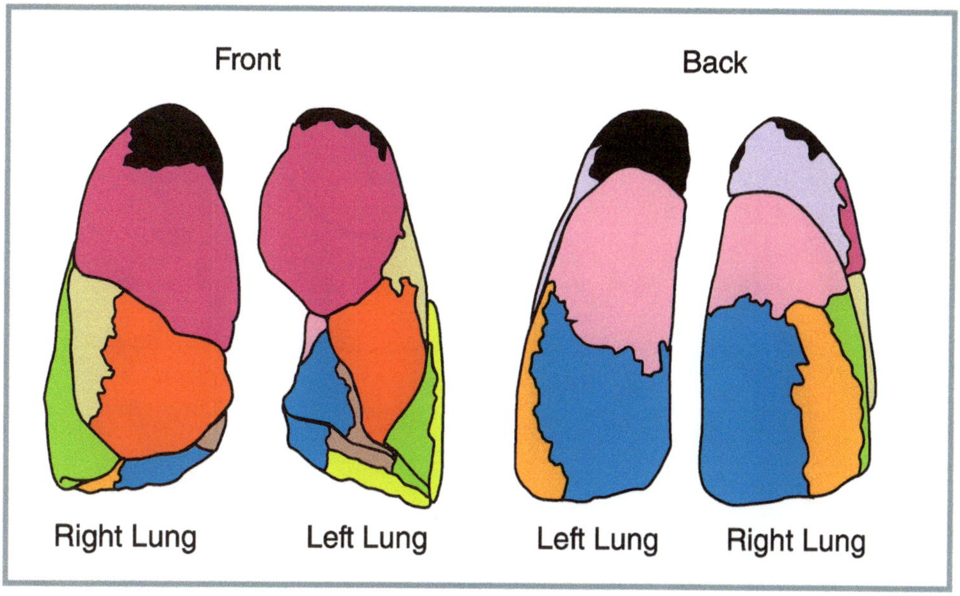

THORAX

Lung Segments

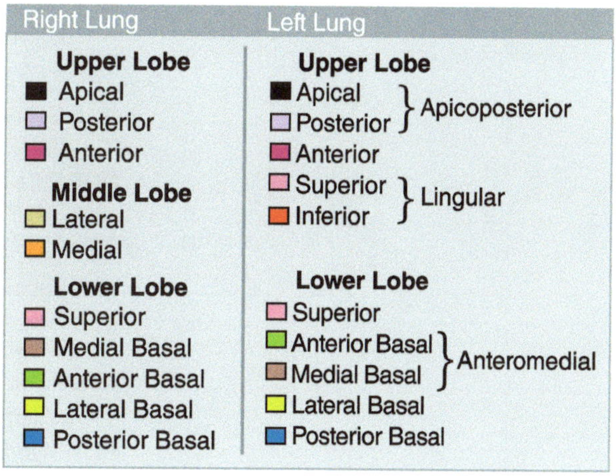

Adapted and modified from Mountain CF and Dresler CM.

* *Mountain CF and Dresler CM. Regional lymph node classification for lung cancer staging. Chest 1997;111:1718–23.*

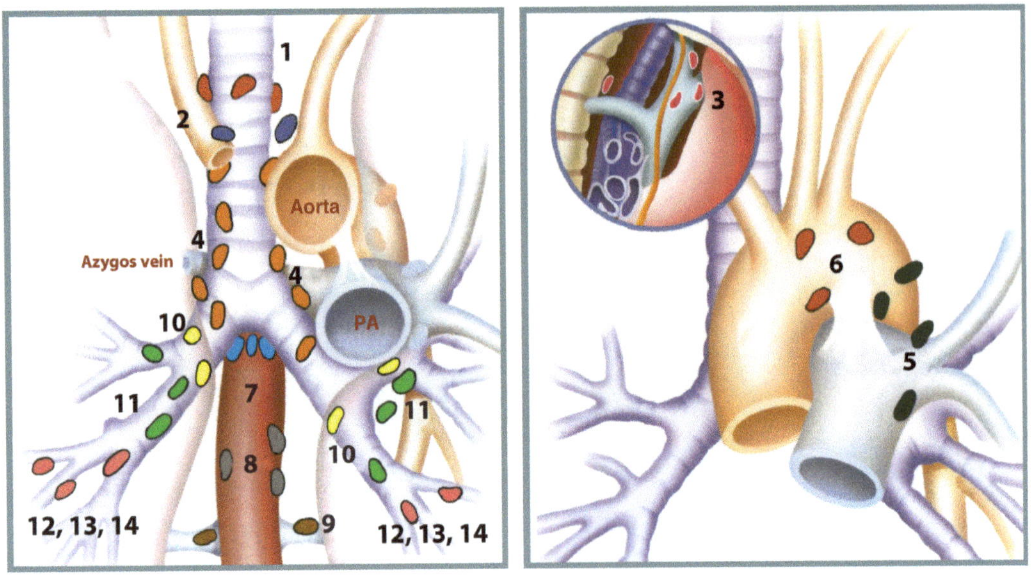

Upper Mediastinal Lymph Nodes

- 1 Upper Mediastinal
- 2 Upper Paratracheal
- 3 Retrotracheal
- 4 Lower paratracheal *(including azygos lymph nodes)*

Aortic Lymph Nodes

- 5 Subaortic *(Aortico-pulmonary window)*
- 6 Para-aortic *(descending aorta and phrenic)*

Lower Mediastinal Lymph Nodes

- 7 Subcarinal
- 8 Para-esophageal *(below the carina)*
- 9 Pulmonary ligament
- 10 Hilar
- 11 Interlober
- 12 Lober
- 13 Segmental
- 14 Subsegmental

Adapted and modified from Mountain CF and Dresler CM.

* *Mountain CF and Dresler CM. Regional lymph node classification for lung cancer staging. Chest 1997;111:1718–23.*

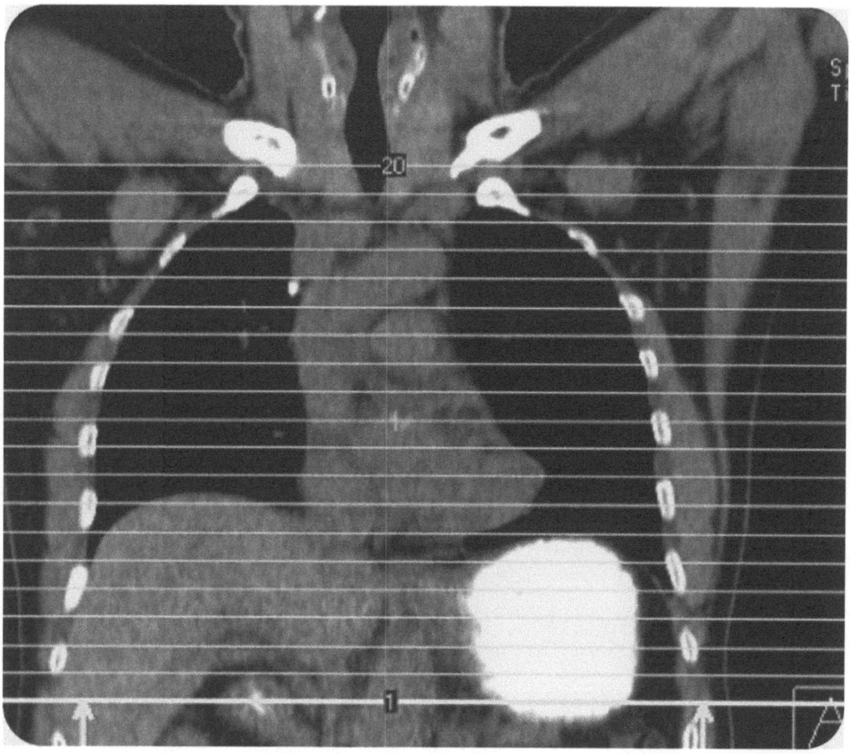

2 ThoraxConsecutive sections were obtained with 3-mm slice thickness and without intravenous contrast. Computed Tomography (CT) images were shown both with mediastinal and lung window settings. Positron Emission Tomography (PET) scintigraphic and CT images obtained from the same level were given side to side for comparison. All anatomic structures in an image were numbered and given in the explanation section at the bottom of the page. Vertebral levels were marked on each vertebra.

Picture 1

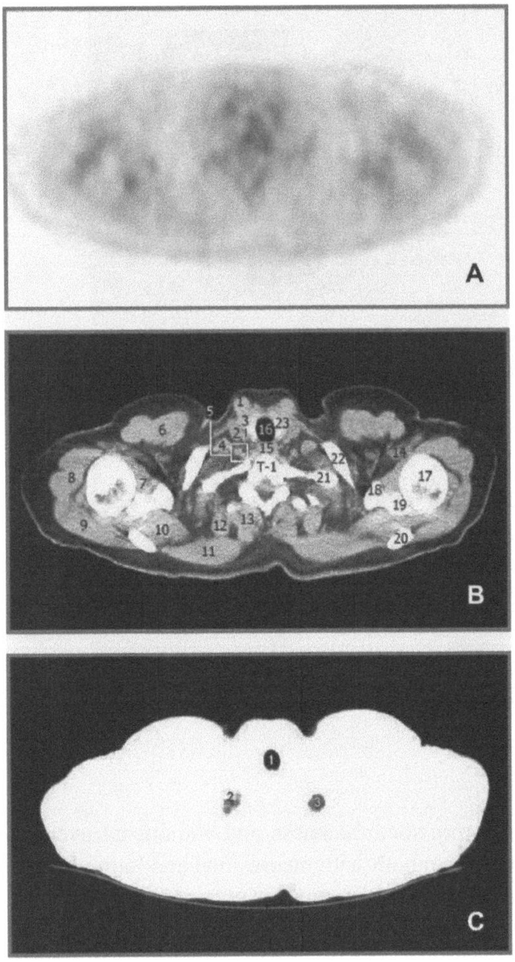

Picture 2

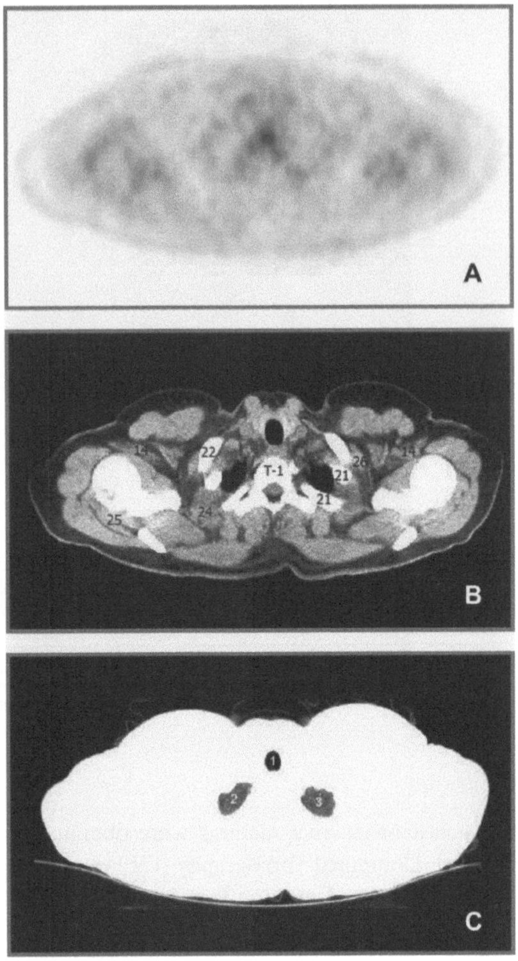

Keys

1. Sternocleidomastoid, sternal head
2. Right internal jugular vein
3. Right common carotid artery
4. Right subclavian artery
5. Vertebral artery and vein
6. Pectoralis major
7. Subscapularis
8. Latissimus dorsi
9. Deltoideus
10. Supraspinatus
11. Trapezius
12. Rhomboideus
13. Erector spinae
14. Axillary artery and vein
15. Oesophagus
16. Trachea
17. Head of humerus
18. Coracoid process
19. Glenoid cavity
20. Spine of scapula
21. 1st rib
22. Clavicle
23. Thyroid gland, left lobe
24. Levator scapulae
25. Supraspinatus
26. Subclavius

Lung parenchymal window

1. Trachea
2. Apical segment, right lung superior lobe
3. Apicoposterior segment, left lung superior lobe

Picture 3

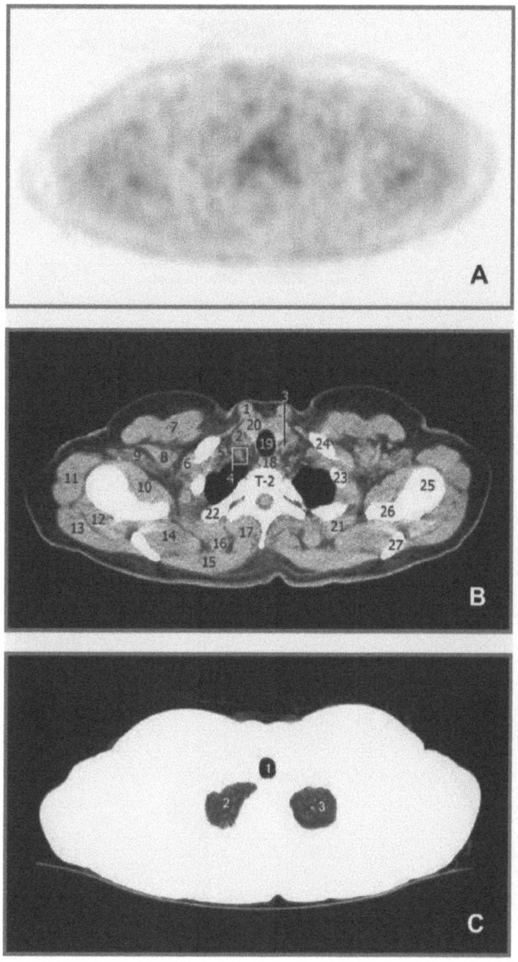

Picture 4

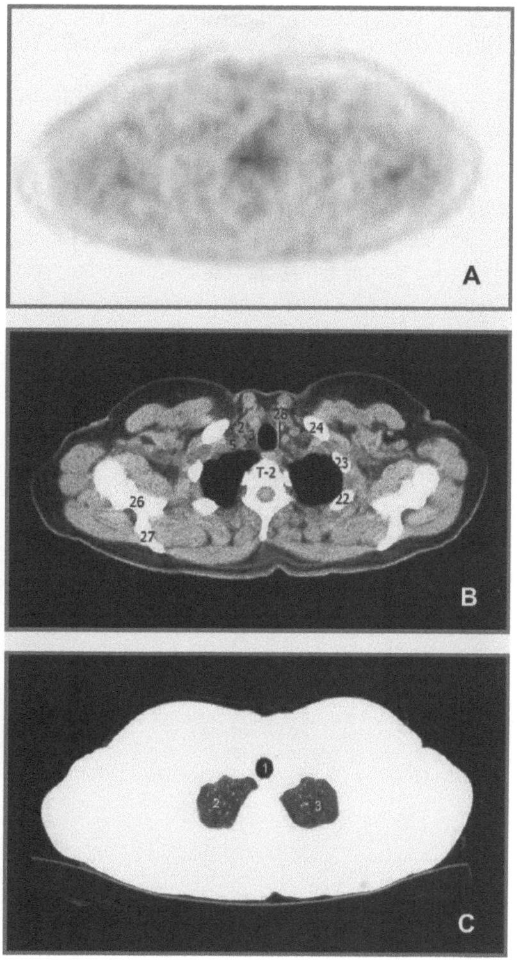

Keys

1. Sternocleidomastoid, sternal head
2. Right internal jugular vein
3. Left common carotid artery
4. Vertebral artery and vein
5. Subclavian artery
6. Subclavius
7. Pectoralis major
8. Pectoralis minor
9. Axillary artery and vein
10. Subscapularis
11. Latissimus dorsi
12. Infraspinatus
13. Deltoideus
14. Supraspinatus
15. Trapezius
16. Rhomboideus
17. Erector spinae
18. Oesophagus
19. Trachea
20. Thyroid gland, right lobe
21. Levator scapulae
22. 2nd rib
23. 1st rib
24. Clavicle
25. Neck of humerus
26. Neck of scapula
27. Spine of scapula
28. Thoracic duct

Lung parenchymal window

1. Trachea
2. Apical segment, right lung superior lobe
3. Apicoposterior segment, left lung superior lobe

Picture 5

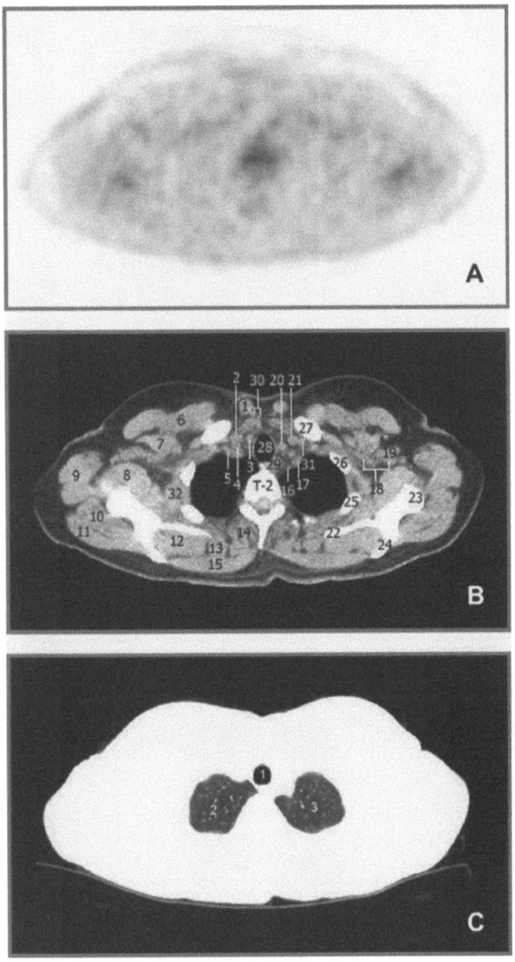

Picture 6

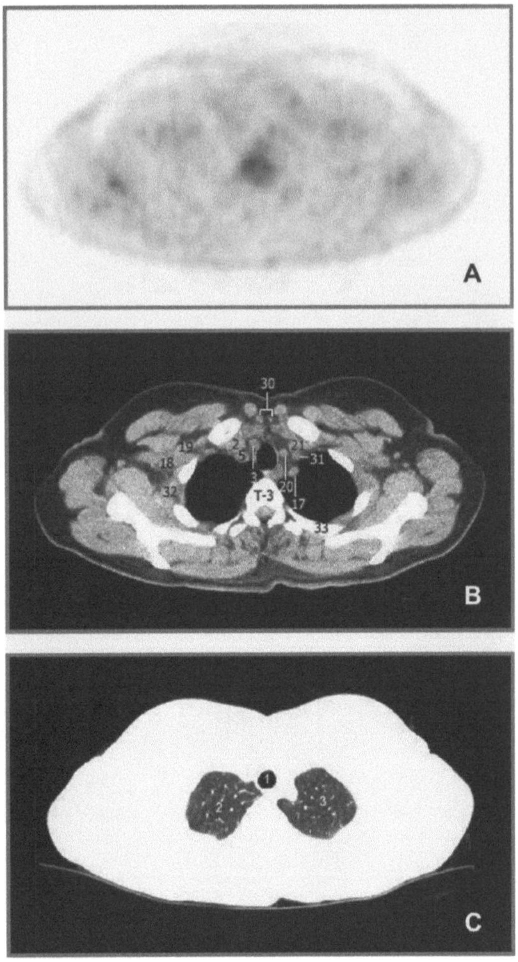

Keys

1. Sternocleidomastoid, sternal head
2. Right brachiocephalic vein
3. Right common carotid artery
4. Right subclavian vein
5. Right subclavian artery
6. Pectoralis major
7. Pectoralis minor
8. Subscapularis
9. Latissimus dorsi
10. Infraspinatus
11. Deltoideus
12. Supraspinatus
13. Rhomboideus
14. Erector spinae
15. Trapezius
16. Thoracic duct
17. Left subclavian artery
18. Axillary artery
19. Axillary vein
20. Left common carotid artery
21. Left brachiocephalic vein
22. Scapula, medial border
23. Infraglenoid tubercle
24. Spine of scapula
25. 2nd rib
26. 1st rib
27. Clavicle, sternal end
28. Trachea
29. Oesophagus
30. Anterior jugular vein
31. Left subclavian vein
32. Serratus anterior
33. 3rd rib

Lung parenchymal window

1. Trachea
2. Apical segment, right lung superior lobe
3. Apicoposterior segment, left lung superior lobe

Picture 7

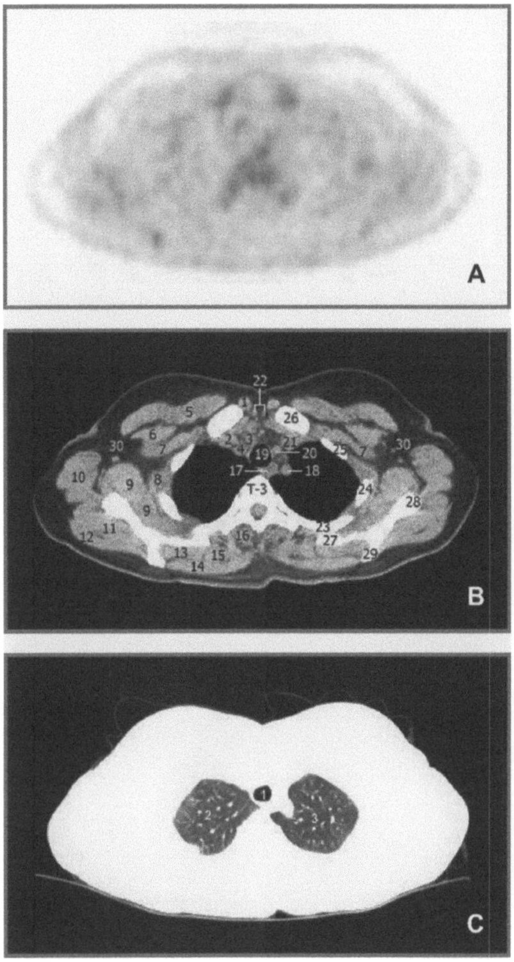

Picture 8

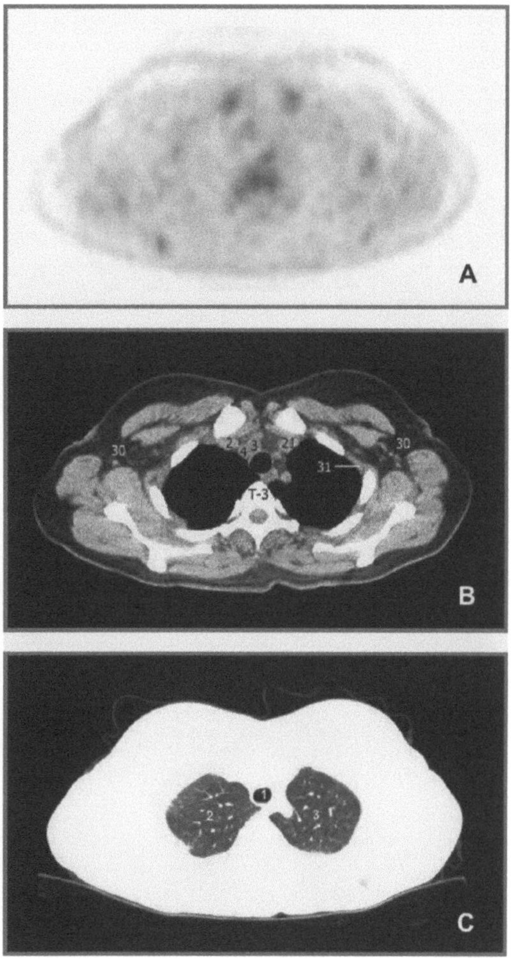

Keys

1. Sternocleidomastoid, sternal head
2. Right brachiocephalic vein
3. Right common carotid artery
4. Right subclavian artery
5. Pectoralis major
6. Pectoralis minor
7. Axillary vein
8. Serratus anterior
9. Subscapularis
10. Latissimus dorsi
11. Infraspinatus
12. Deltoideus
13. Supraspinatus
14. Trapezius
15. Rhomboideus
16. Erector spinae
17. Oesophagus
18. Left subclavian artery
19. Trachea
20. Left common carotid artery
21. Left brachiocephalic vein
22. Anterior jugular vein
23. 3rd rib
24. 2nd rib
25. 1st rib
26. Clavicle, sternal end
27. Scapula, medial border
28. Infraglenoid tubercle
29. Spine of scapula
30. Axillary fossa
31. Intercostal muscles

Lung parenchymal window

1. Trachea
2. Apical segment, right lung superior lobe
3. Apicoposterior segment, left lung superior lobe

Picture 9

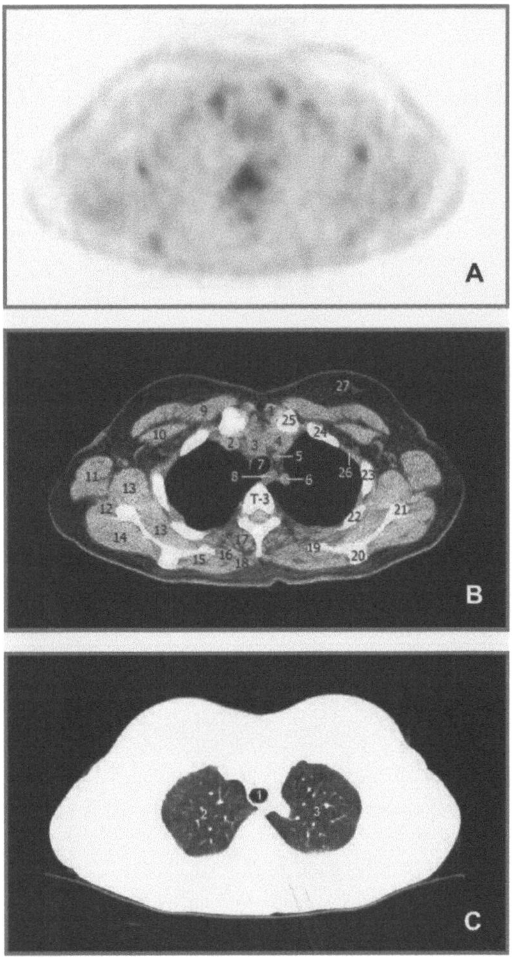

Picture 10

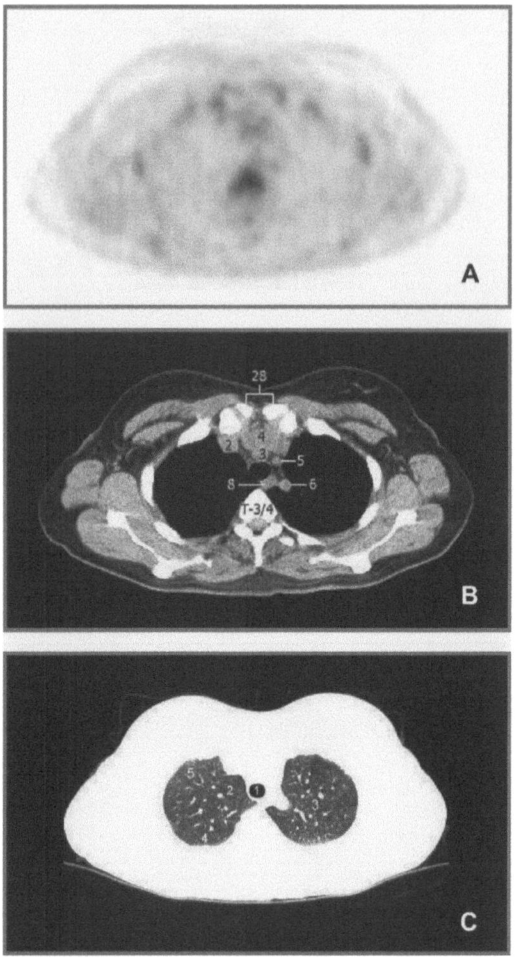

Keys

1. Sternocleidomastoid, sternal head
2. Right brachiocephalic vein
3. Brachiocephalic trunk
4. Left brachiocephalic vein
5. Left common carotid artery
6. Left subclavian artery
7. Trachea
8. Oesophagus
9. Pectoralis major
10. Pectoralis minor
11. Latissimus dorsi
12. Teres minor
13. Subscapularis
14. Infraspinatus
15. Supraspinatus
16. Rhomboideus
17. Erector spinae
18. Trapezius
19. Scapula, medial border
20. Spine of scapula
21. Scapula, lateral border
22. 3rd rib
23. 2nd rib
24. 1st rib
25. Clavicle, sternal end
26. Intercostal muscles
27. Breast
28. Manubrium of sternum

Lung parenchymal window

1. Trachea
2. Apical segment, right lung superior lobe
3. Apicoposterior segment, left lung superior lobe
4. Posterior segment, right lung superior lobe
5. Anterior segment, right lung superior lobe

Picture 11

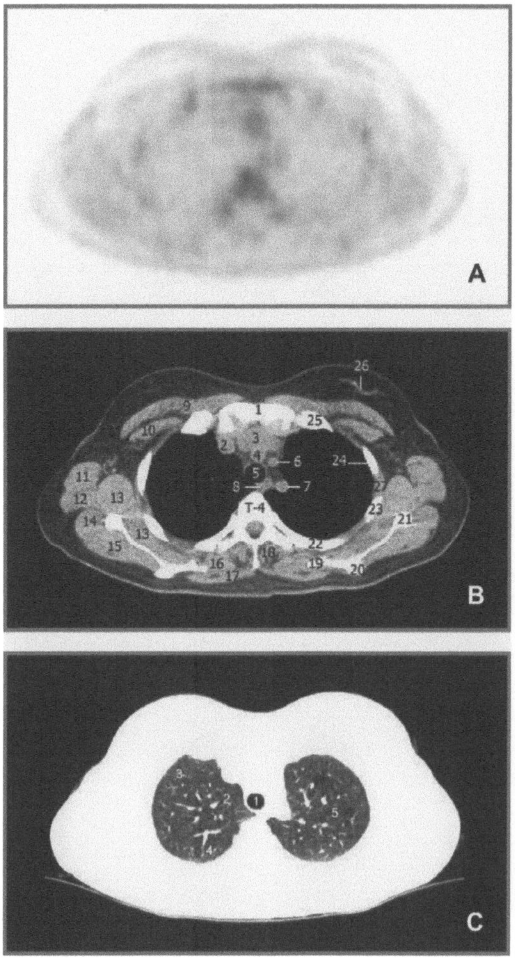

Picture 12

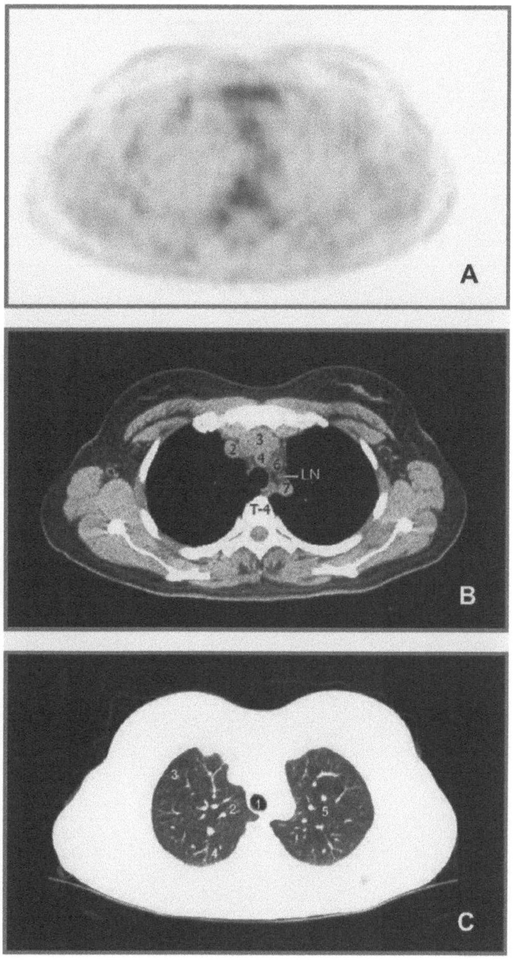

Keys

1. Manubrium of sternum
2. Right brachiocephalic vein
3. Left brachiocephalic vein
4. Brachiocephalic trunk
5. Trachea
6. Left common carotid artery
7. Left subclavian artery
8. Oesophagus
9. Pectoralis major
10. Pectoralis minor
11. Latissimus dorsi
12. Teres major
13. Subscapularis
14. Teres minor
15. Infraspinatus
16. Rhomboideus
17. Trapezius
18. Erector spinae
19. Scapula, medial border
20. Spine of scapula
21. Scapula, lateral border
22. 4th rib
23. 3rd rib
24. 2nd rib
25. 1st rib
26. Breast
27. Serratus anterior

LN Lymph node

Lung parenchymal window

1. Trachea
2. Apical segment, right lung superior lobe,
3. Anterior segment, right lung superior lobe
4. Posterior segment, right lung superior lobe
5. Apicoposterior segment, left lung superior lobe

Picture 13

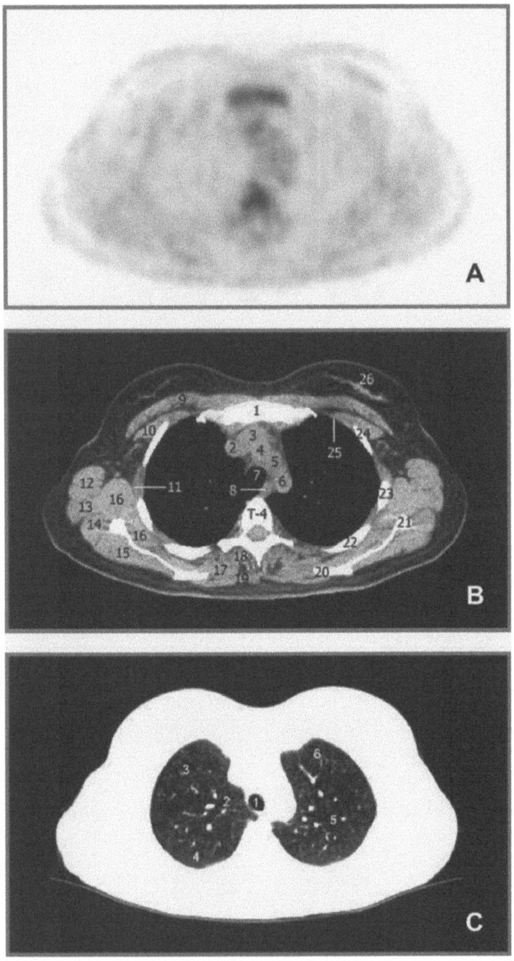

Picture 14

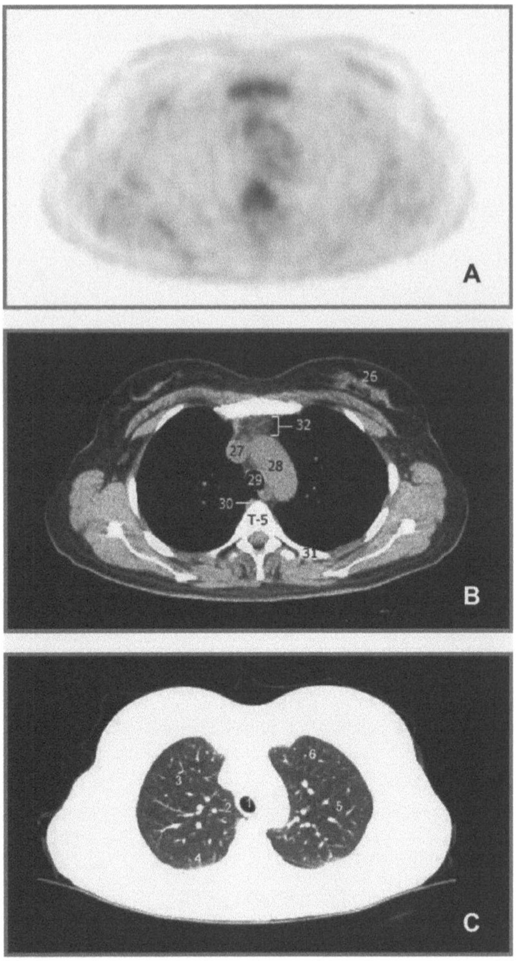

Keys

1. Manubrium of sternum
2. Right brachiocephalic vein
3. Left brachiocephalic vein
4. Brachiocephalic trunk
5. Left common carotid artery
6. Left subclavian artery
7. Trachea
8. Oesophagus
9. Pectoralis major
10. Pectoralis minor
11. Serratus anterior
12. Latissimus dorsi
13. Teres major
14. Teres minor
15. Infraspinatus
16. Subscapularis
17. Rhomboideus
18. Erector spinae
19. Trapezius
20. Scapula, medial border
21. Scapula, lateral border
22. 4th rib
23. 3rd rib
24. 2nd rib
25. Intercostal muscles
26. Breast
27. Superior caval vein
28. Aortic arch
29. Tracheal bifurcation
30. Azygos vein
31. 5th rib
32. Anterior mediastinal fat pad

Lung parenchymal window

1. Trachea
2. Apical segment, right lung superior lobe
3. Anterior segment, right lung superior lobe
4. Posterior segment, right lung superior lobe
5. Apicoposterior segment, left lung superior lobe
6. Anterior segment, left lung superior lobe

Picture 15

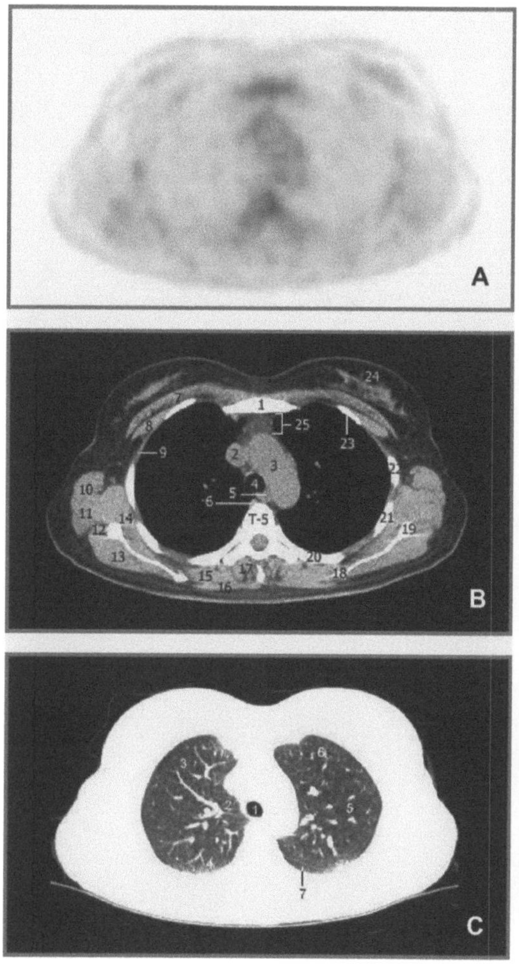

Picture 16

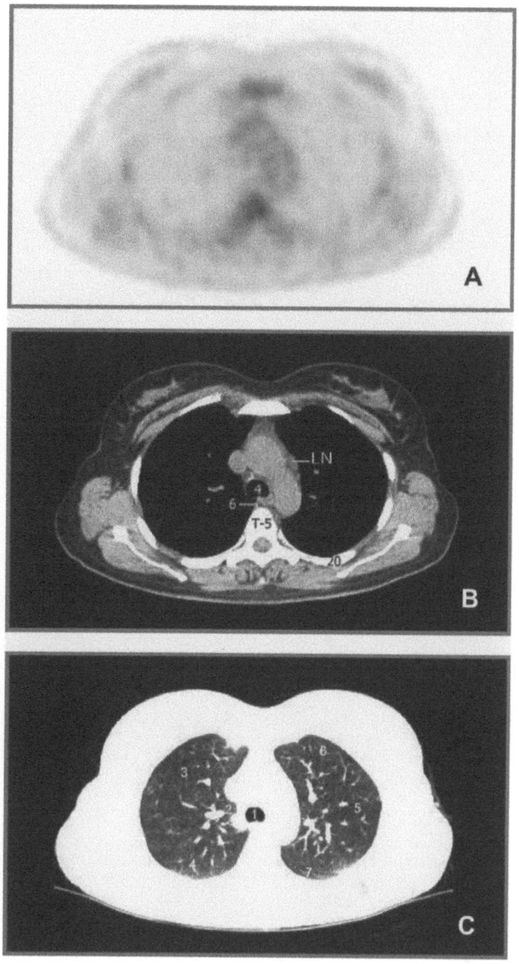

Keys

1. Manubrium of sternum
2. Superior caval vein
3. Aortic arch
4. Tracheal bifurcation
5. Oesophagus
6. Azygos vein
7. Pectoralis major
8. Pectoralis minor
9. Intercostal muscles
10. Latissimus dorsi
11. Teres major
12. Teres minor
13. Infraspinatus
14. Subscapularis
15. Rhomboideus
16. Trapezius
17. Erector spinae
18. Scapula, medial border
19. Scapula, lateral border
20. 5th rib
21. 4th rib
22. 3rd rib
23. 2nd rib
24. Breast
25. Anterior mediastinal fat pad

LN Lymph node

Lung parenchymal window

1. Trachea
2. Apical segment, right lung superior lobe
3. Anterior segment, right lung superior lobe
4. Posterior segment, right lung superior lobe
5. Apicoposterior segment, left lung superior lobe
6. Anterior segment, left lung superior lobe
7. Superior segment, left lung inferior lobe

Picture 17

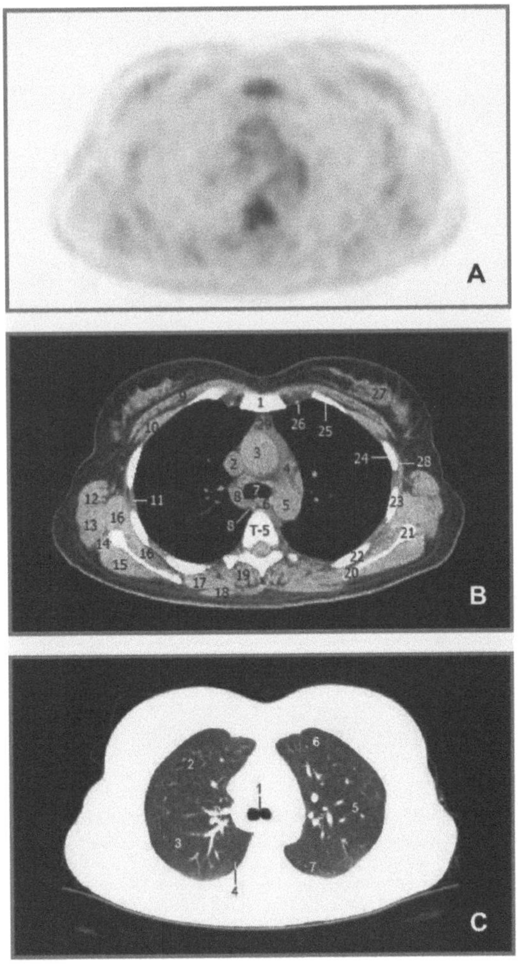

Picture 18

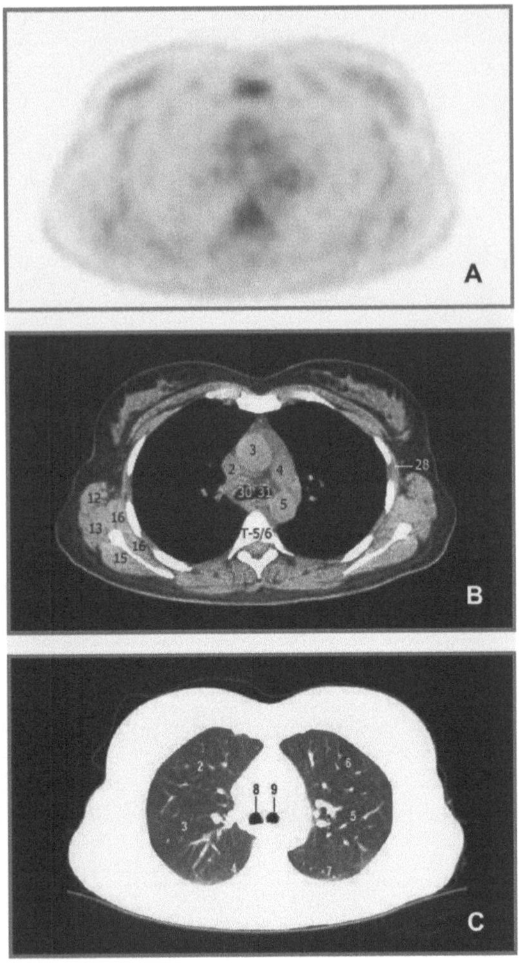

Keys

1. Sternum
2. Superior caval vein
3. Ascending aorta
4. Aortopulmonary window
5. Thoracic aorta
6. Oesophagus
7. Tracheal bifurcation
8. Azygos vein
9. Pectoralis major
10. Pectoralis minor
11. Intercostal muscles
12. Latissimus dorsi
13. Teres major
14. Teres minor
15. Infraspinatus
16. Subscapularis
17. Rhomboideus
18. Trapezius
19. Erector spinae
20. Scapula, medial border
21. Scapula, lateral border
22. 5th rib
23. 4th rib
24. 3rd rib
25. 2nd rib
26. Internal thoracic artery
27. Breast
28. Serratus anterior
29. Anterior mediastinal fat pad
30. Right main bronchus
31. Left main bronchus

Lung parenchymal window

1. Carina (bifurcation of the trachea)
2. Anterior segment, right lung superior lobe
3. Posterior segment, right lung superior lobe
4. Superior segment, right lung inferior lobe
5. Apicoposterior segment, left lung superior lobe
6. Anterior segment, left lung superior lobe
7. Superior segment, left lung inferior lobe
8. Right main bronchus
9. Left main bronchus

Picture 19

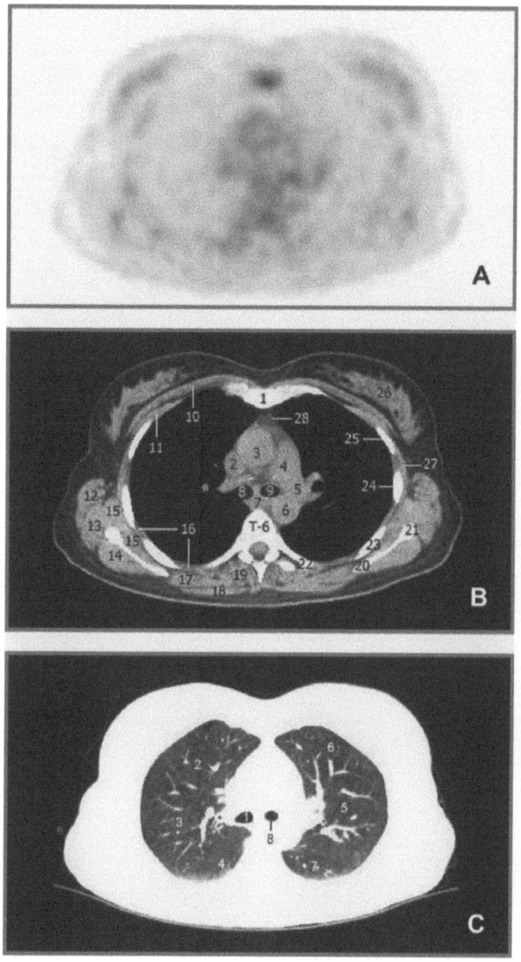

Picture 20

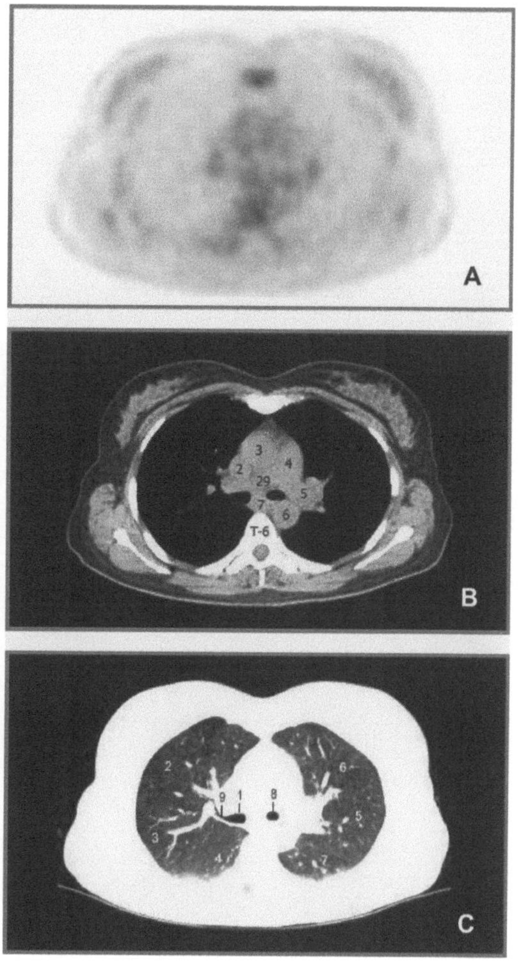

Keys

1. Sternum
2. Superior caval vein
3. Ascending aorta
4. Pulmonary trunk
5. Left pulmonary artery
6. Thoracic aorta
7. Oesophagus
8. Right main bronchus
9. Left main bronchus
10. Pectoralis major
11. Pectoralis minor
12. Latissimus dorsi
13. Teres major
14. Infraspinatus
15. Subscapularis
16. Intercostal muscles
17. Rhomboideus
18. Trapezius
19. Erector spinae
20. Scapula, medial border
21. Scapula, lateral border
22. 6th rib
23. 5th rib
24. 4th rib
25. 3rd rib
26. Breast
27. Serratus anterior
28. Anterior mediastinal fat pad
29. Right pulmonary artery

Lung parenchymal window

1. Right main bronchus
2. Anterior segment, right lung superior lobe
3. Posterior segment, right lung superior lobe
4. Superior segment, right lung inferior lobe
5. Apicoposterior segment, left lung superior lobe
6. Anterior segment, left lung superior lobe
7. Superior segment, left lung inferior lobe
8. Left main bronchus
9. Right superior lobar bronchus

Picture 21

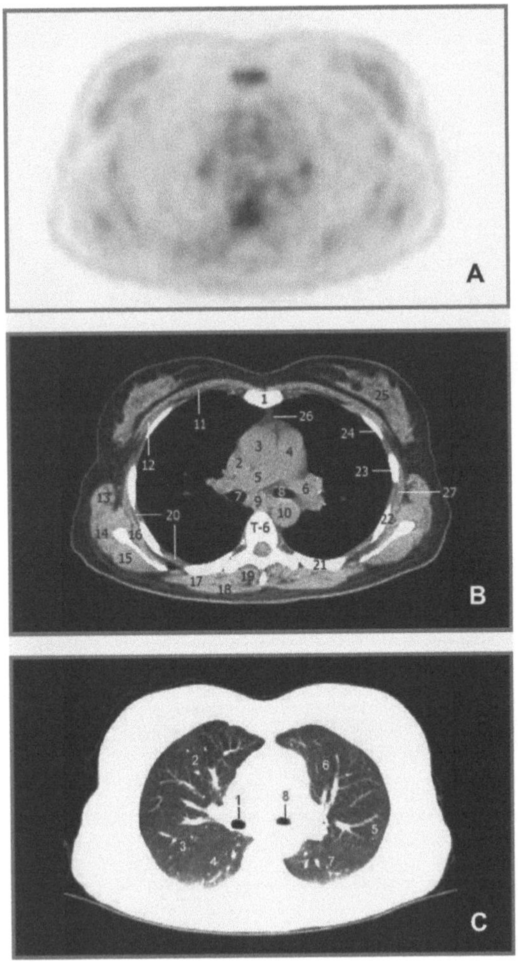

Picture 22

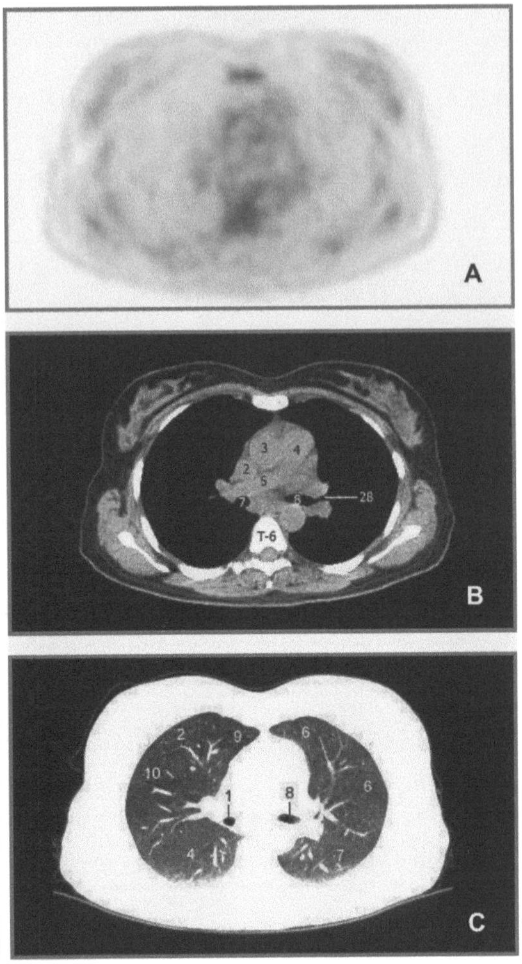

Keys

1. Sternum
2. Superior caval vein
3. Ascending aorta
4. Pulmonary trunk
5. Right pulmonary artery
6. Left pulmonary artery
7. Right main bronchus
8. Left main bronchus
9. Oesophagus
10. Thoracic aorta
11. Pectoralis major
12. Pectoralis minor
13. Latissimus dorsi
14. Teres major
15. Infraspinatus
16. Subscapularis
17. Rhomboideus
18. Trapezius
19. Erector spinae
20. Intercostal muscles
21. 6th rib
22. 5th rib
23. 4th rib
24. 3rd rib
25. Breast
26. Anterior mediastinal fat pad
27. Serratus anterior
28. Left superior lobar bronchus

Lung parenchymal window

1. Right intermediate bronchus
2. Anterior segment, right lung superior lobe
3. Posterior segment, right lung superior lobe
4. Superior segment, right lung inferior lobe
5. Apicoposterior segment, left lung superior lobe
6. Anterior segment, left lung superior lobe
7. Superior segment, left lung inferior lobe
8. Left main bronchus
9. Medial segment, right lung middle lobe
10. Lateral segment, right lung middle lobe

Picture 23

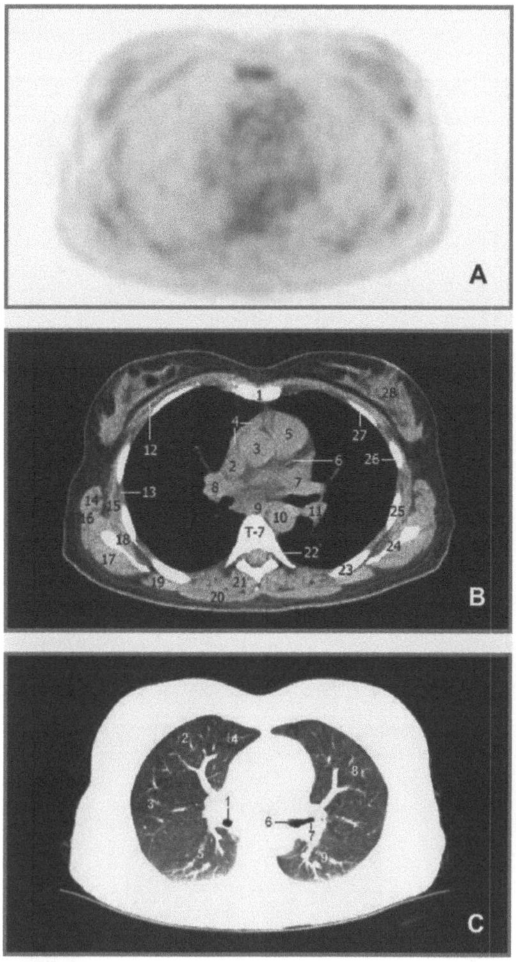

Picture 24

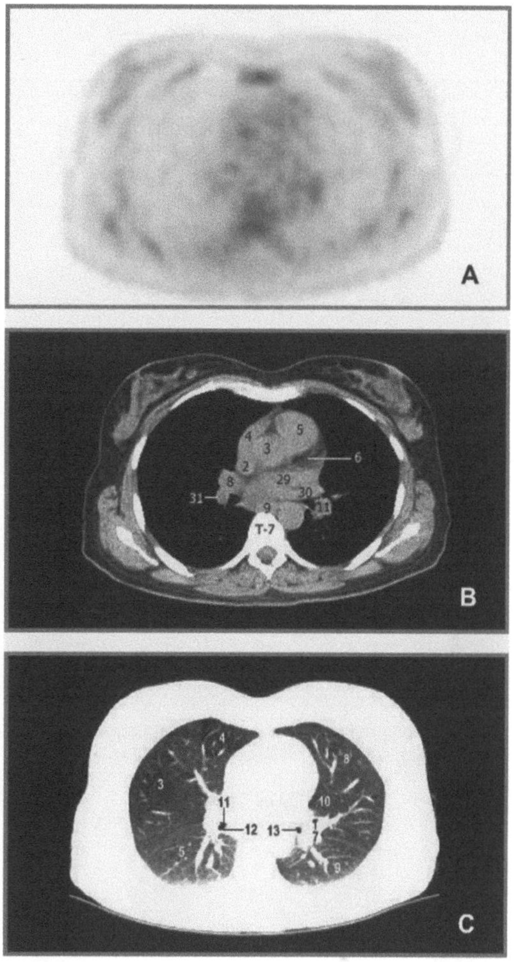

Keys

1. Sternum
2. Superior caval vein
3. Ascending aorta
4. Right auricle
5. Pulmonary trunk
6. Left coronary artery
7. Left pulmonary artery
8. Right superior pulmonary artery
9. Oesophagus
10. Thoracic aorta
11. Left inferior pulmonary artery
12. Pectoralis major
13. Intercostal muscles
14. Latissimus dorsi
15. Serratus anterior
16. Teres major
17. Infraspinatus
18. Subscapularis
19. Rhomboideus
20. Trapezius
21. Erector spinae
22. 7th rib
23. 6th rib
24. Scapula
25. 5th rib
26. 4th rib
27. 3rd rib
28. Breast
29. Left atrium
30. Left superior pulmonary vein
31. Right superior pulmonary vein

Lung parenchymal window

1. Right intermediate bronchus
2. Anterior segment, right lung superior lobe
3. Lateral segment, right lung middle lobe
4. Medial segment, right lung middle lobe
5. Superior segment, right lung inferior lobe
6. Left main bronchus
7. Left superior lobar bronchus
8. Anterior segment, left lung superior lobe
9. Superior segment, left lung inferior lobe
10. Superior lingular segment, left lung superior lobe
11. Right middle lobar bronchus
12. Right inferior lobar bronchus
13. Left inferior lobar bronchus

Picture 25

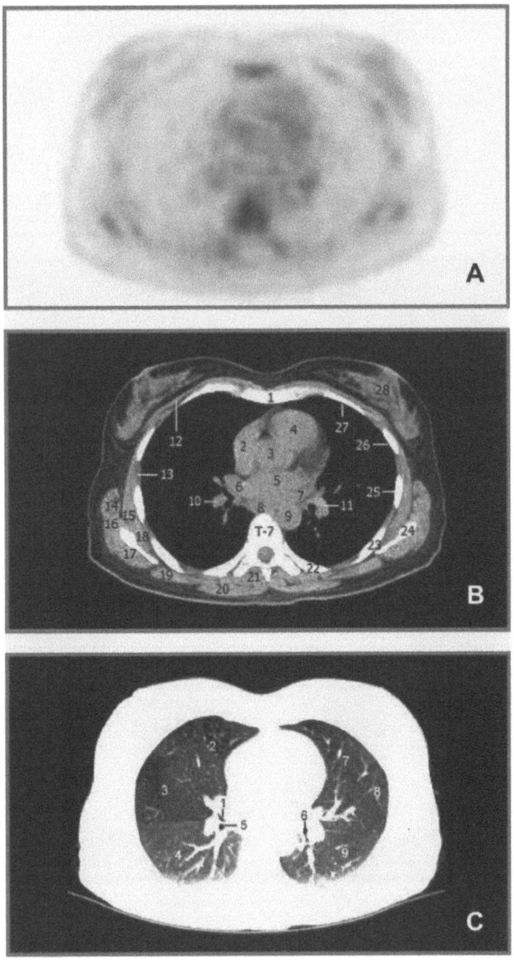

Picture 26

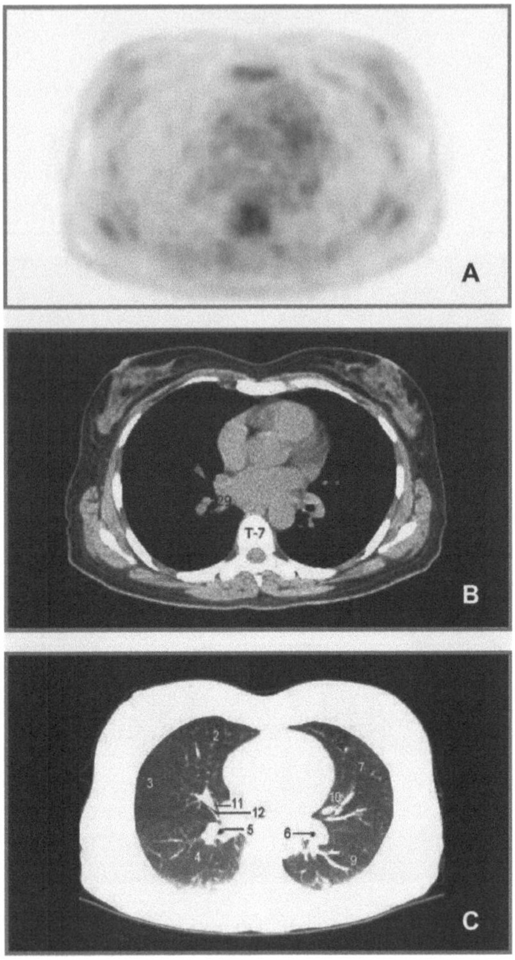

Keys

1. Sternum
2. Right atrium
3. Ascending aorta
4. Infundibulum
5. Left atrium
6. Right superior pulmonary vein
7. Left superior pulmonary vein
8. Oesophagus
9. Thoracic aorta
10. Right inferior pulmonary artery
11. Left inferior pulmonary artery
12. Pectoralis major
13. Intercostal muscles
14. Latissimus dorsi
15. Serratus anterior
16. Teres major
17. Infraspinatus
18. Subscapularis
19. Rhomboideus
20. Trapezius
21. Erector spinae
22. 7th rib
23. 6th rib
24. Scapula
25. 5th rib
26. 4th rib
27. 3rd rib
28. Breast
29. Right inferior pulmonary vein

Lung parenchymal window

1. Right middle lobar bronchus
2. Medial segment, right lung middle lobe
3. Lateral segment, right lung middle lobe
4. Superior segment, right lung inferior lobe
5. Right inferior lobar bronchus
6. Left inferior lobar bronchus
7. Superior lingular segment, left lung superior lobe
8. Anterior segment, left lung superior lobe
9. Superior segment, left lung inferior lobe
10. Inferior lingular segment, left lung superior lobe
11. Medial segmental bronchus of right lung middle lobe
12. Lateral segmental bronchus of right lung middle lobe

Picture 27

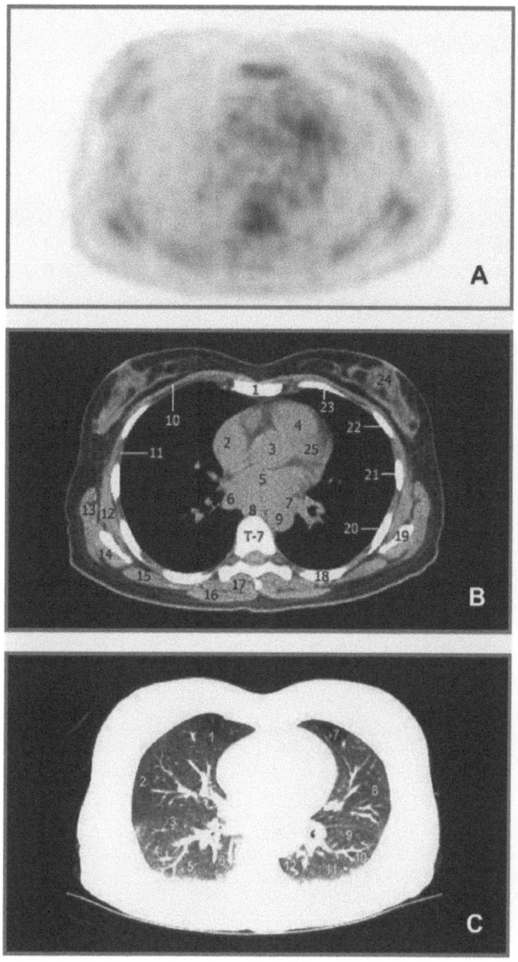

Picture 28

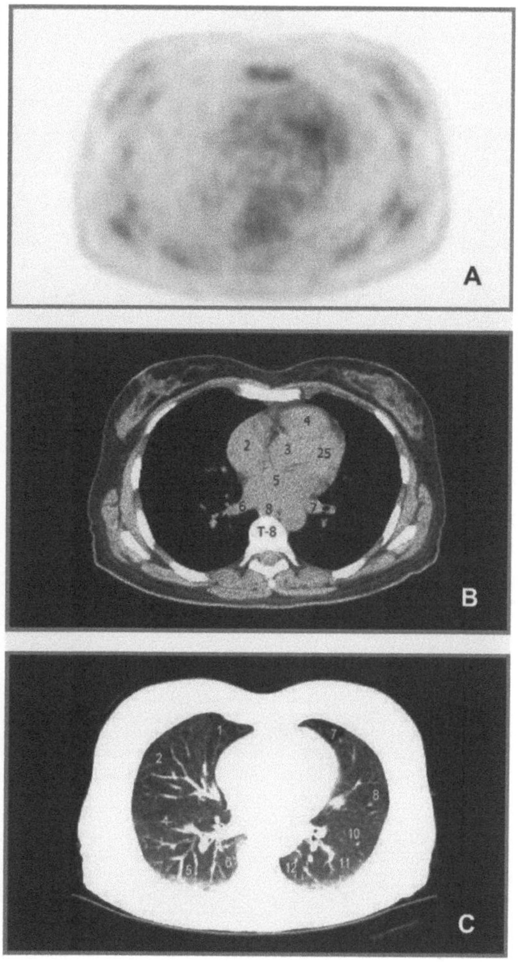

Keys

1. Sternum
2. Right atrium
3. Aortic bulb
4. Right ventricle
5. Left atrium
6. Right inferior pulmonary vein
7. Left inferior pulmonary vein
8. Oesophagus
9. Thoracic aorta
10. Pectoralis major
11. Intercostal muscles
12. Serratus anterior
13. Latissimus dorsi
14. Infraspinatus
15. Rhomboideus
16. Trapezius
17. Erector spinae
18. 7th rib
19. Scapula
20. 6th rib
21. 5th rib
22. 4th rib
23. 3rd rib
24. Breast
25. Left ventricle

Lung parenchymal window

1. Medial segment, right lung middle lobe
2. Lateral segment, right lung middle lobe
3. Superior segment, right lung inferior lobe
4. Anterior basal segment, right lung inferior lobe
5. Lateral basal segment, right lung inferior lobe
6. Posterior basal segment, right lung inferior lobe
7. Superior lingular segment, left lung superior lobe
8. Inferior lingular segment, left lung superior lobe
9. Superior segment, left lung inferior lobe
10. Anterior basal segment, left lung inferior lobe
11. Lateral basal segment, left lung inferior lobe
12. Posterior basal segment, left lung inferior lobe

Picture 29

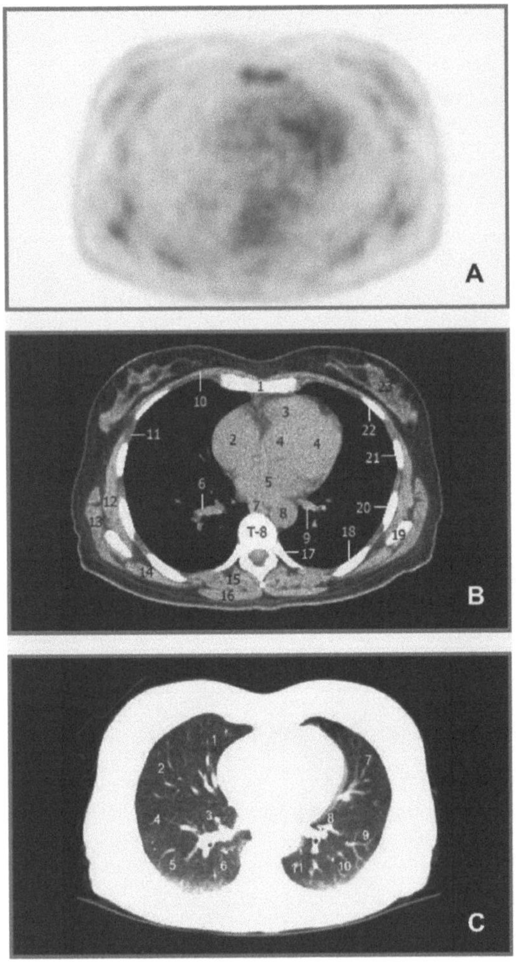

Picture 30

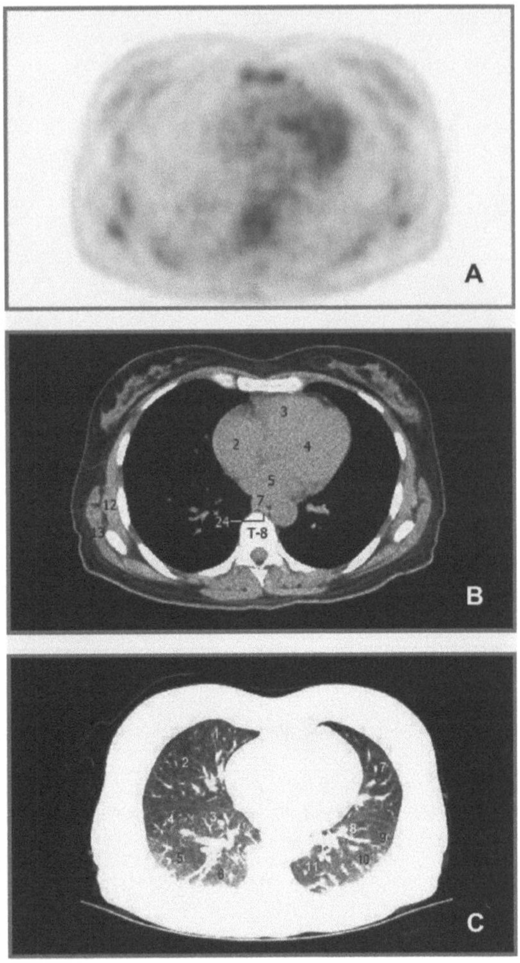

Keys

1. Sternum
2. Right atrium
3. Right ventricle
4. Left ventricle
5. Left atrium
6. Right inferior pulmonary vein
7. Oesophagus
8. Thoracic aorta
9. Left inferior pulmonary vein
10. Pectoralis major
11. Intercostal muscles
12. Serratus anterior
13. Latissimus dorsi
14. Rhomboideus
15. Erector spinae
16. Trapezius
17. 8th rib
18. 7th rib
19. Scapula, inferior angle
20. 6th rib
21. 5th rib
22. 4th rib
23. Breast
24. Azygos vein

Lung parenchymal window

1. Medial segment, right lung middle lobe
2. Lateral segment, right lung middle lobe
3. Medial basal segment, right lung inferior lobe
4. Anterior basal segment, right lung inferior lobe
5. Lateral basal segment, right lung inferior lobe
6. Posterior basal segment, right lung inferior lobe
7. Inferior lingular segment, left lung superior lobe
8. Medial basal segment, left lung inferior lobe
9. Anterior basal segment, left lung inferior lobe
10. Lateral basal segment, left lung inferior lobe
11. Posterior basal segment, left lung inferior lobe

Picture 31

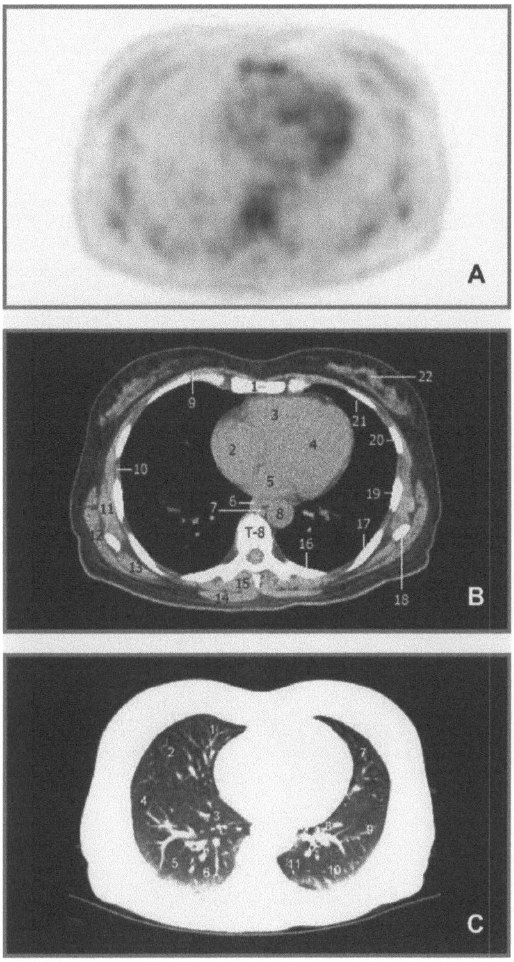

Picture 32

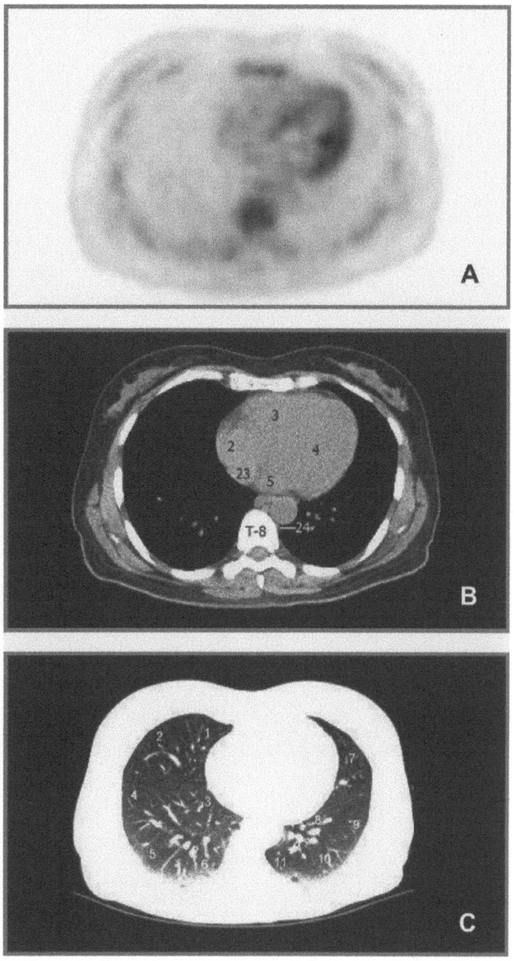

Keys

1. Sternum
2. Right atrium
3. Right ventricle
4. Left ventricle
5. Left atrium
6. Oesophagus
7. Azygos vein
8. Thoracic aorta
9. Pectoralis major
10. Intercostal muscles
11. Serratus anterior
12. Latissimus dorsi
13. Rhomboideus
14. Trapezius
15. Erector spinae
16. 8th rib
17. 7th rib
18. Scapula, inferior angle
19. 6th rib
20. 5th rib
21. 4th rib
22. Breast
23. Inferior caval vein
24. Hemiazygos vein

Lung parenchymal window

1. Medial segment, right lung middle lobe
2. Lateral segment, right lung middle lobe
3. Medial basal segment, right lung inferior lobe
4. Anterior basal segment, right lung inferior lobe
5. Lateral basal segment, right lung inferior lobe
6. Posterior basal segment, right lung inferior lobe
7. Inferior lingular segment, left lung superior lobe
8. Medial basal segment, left lung inferior lobe
9. Anterior basal segment, left lung inferior lobe
10. Lateral basal segment, left lung inferior lobe
11. Posterior basal segment, left lung inferior lobe

Picture 33

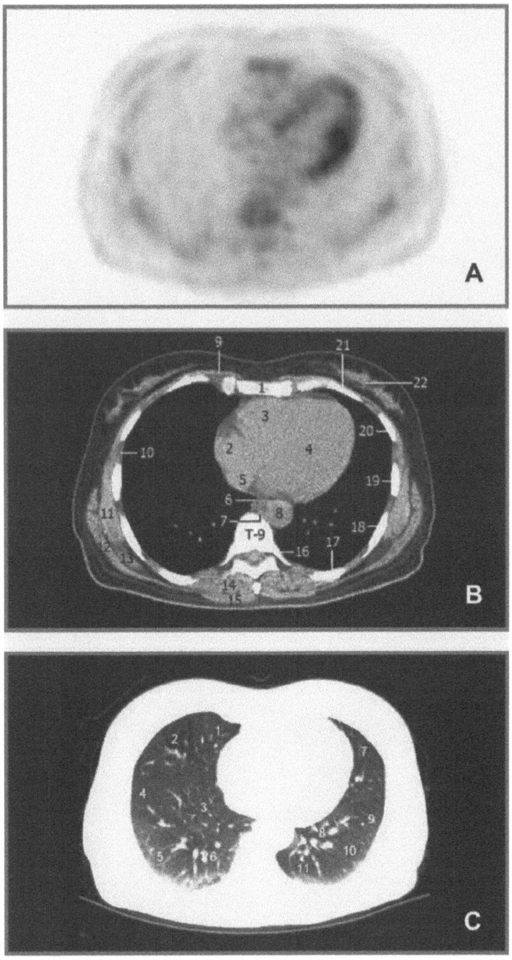

Picture 34

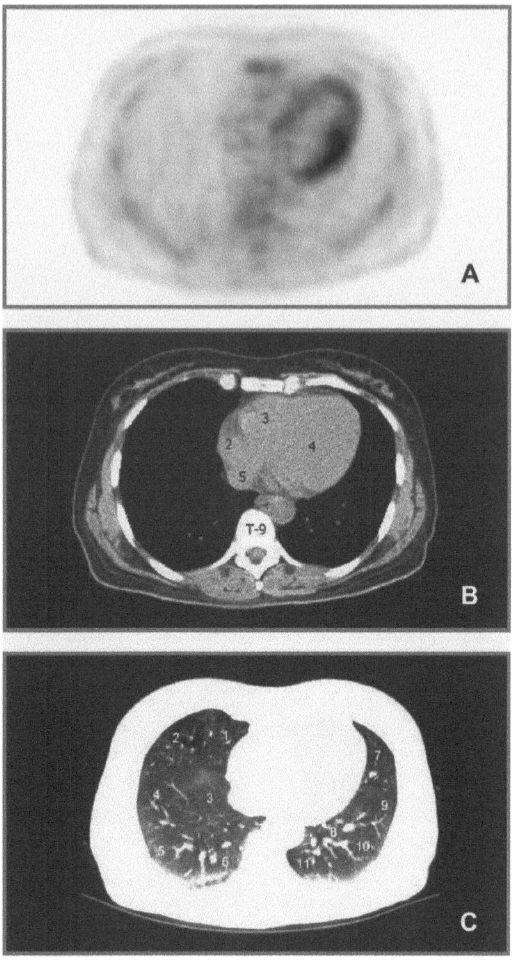

Keys

1. Sternum
2. Right atrium
3. Right ventricle
4. Left ventricle
5. Inferior caval vein
6. Oesophagus
7. Azygos vein
8. Thoracic aorta
9. Pectoralis major
10. Intercostal muscles
11. Serratus anterior
12. Latissimus dorsi
13. Rhomboideus
14. Erector spinae
15. Trapezius
16. 9th rib
17. 8th rib
18. 7th rib
19. 6th rib
20. 5th rib
21. 4th rib
22. Breast

Lung parenchymal window

1. Medial segment, right lung middle lobe
2. Lateral segment, right lung middle lobe
3. Medial basal segment, right lung inferior lobe
4. Anterior basal segment, right lung inferior lobe
5. Lateral basal segment, right lung inferior lobe
6. Posterior basal segment, right lung inferior lobe
7. Inferior lingular segment, left lung superior lobe
8. Medial basal segment, left lung inferior lobe
9. Anterior basal segment, left lung inferior lobe
10. Lateral basal segment, left lung inferior lobe
11. Posterior basal segment, left lung inferior lobe

Picture 35

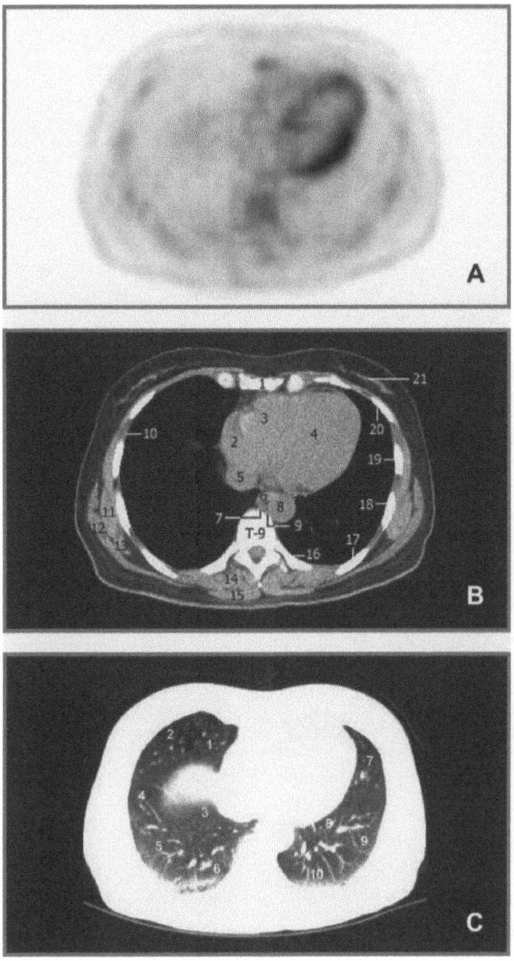

Picture 36

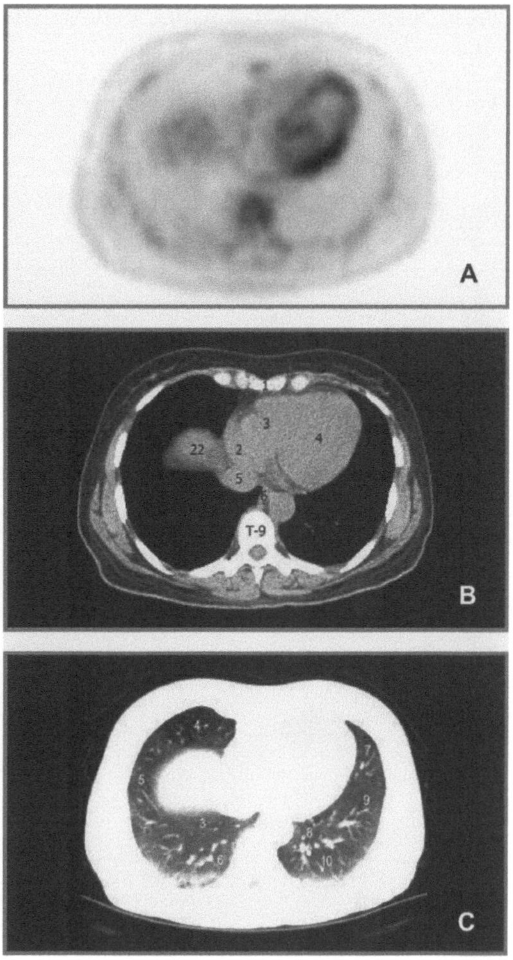

Keys

1. Sternum
2. Right atrium
3. Right ventricle
4. Left ventricle
5. Inferior caval vein
6. Oesophagus
7. Azygos vein
8. Thoracic aorta
9. Thoracic duct
10. Intercostal muscles
11. Serratus anterior
12. Latissimus dorsi
13. Rhomboideus
14. Erector spinae
15. Trapezius
16. 9th rib
17. 8th rib
18. 7th rib
19. 6th rib
20. 5th rib
21. Breast
22. Liver

Lung parenchymal window

1. Medial segment, right lung middle lobe
2. Lateral segment, right lung middle lobe
3. Medial basal segment, right lung inferior lobe
4. Anterior basal segment, right lung inferior lobe
5. Lateral basal segment, right lung inferior lobe
6. Posterior basal segment, right lung inferior lobe
7. Anterior basal segment, left lung inferior lobe
8. Medial basal segment, left lung inferior lobe
9. Lateral basal segment, left lung inferior lobe
10. Posterior basal segment, left lung inferior lobe

Picture 37

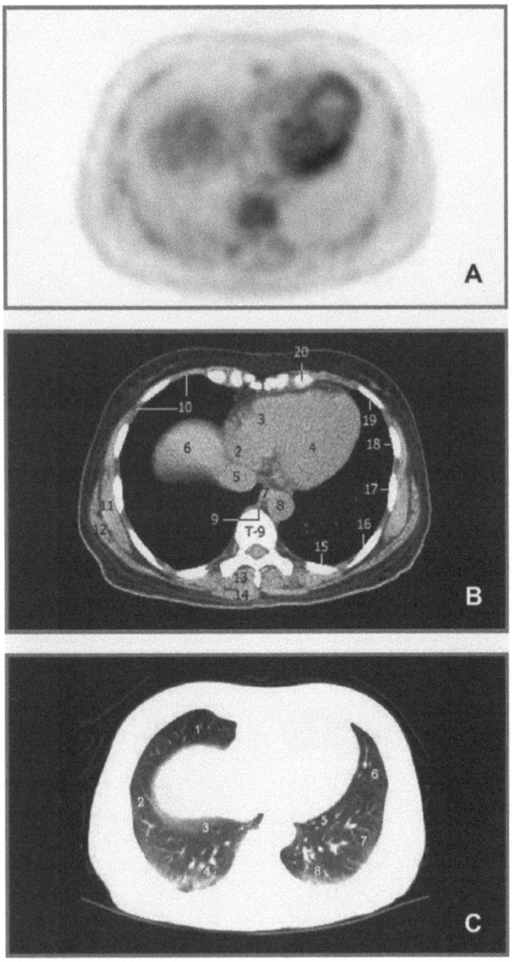

Picture 38

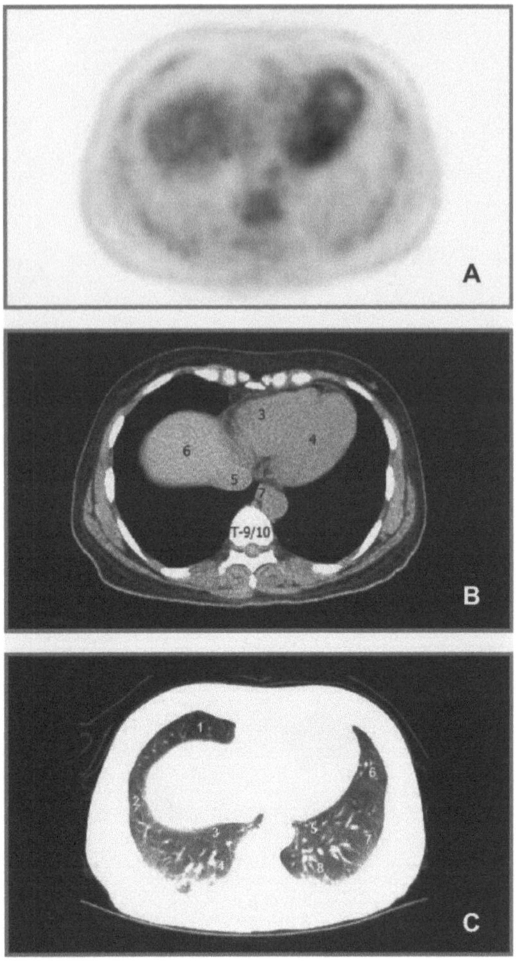

Keys

1. Sternum, xiphoid process
2. Right atrium
3. Right ventricle
4. Left ventricle
5. Inferior caval vein
6. Liver
7. Oesophagus
8. Thoracic aorta
9. Azygos vein
10. Intercostal muscles
11. Serratus anterior
12. Latissimus dorsi
13. Erector spinae
14. Trapezius
15. 9th rib
16. 8th rib
17. 7th rib
18. 6th rib
19. 5th rib
20. Sternocostal joint

Lung parenchymal window

1. Anterior basal segment, right lung inferior lobe
2. Lateral basal segment, right lung inferior lobe
3. Medial basal segment, right lung inferior lobe
4. Posterior basal segment, right lung inferior lobe
5. Medial basal segment, left lung inferior lobe
6. Anterior basal segment, left lung inferior lobe
7. Lateral basal segment, left lung inferior lobe
8. Posterior basal segment, left lung inferior lobe

Picture 39

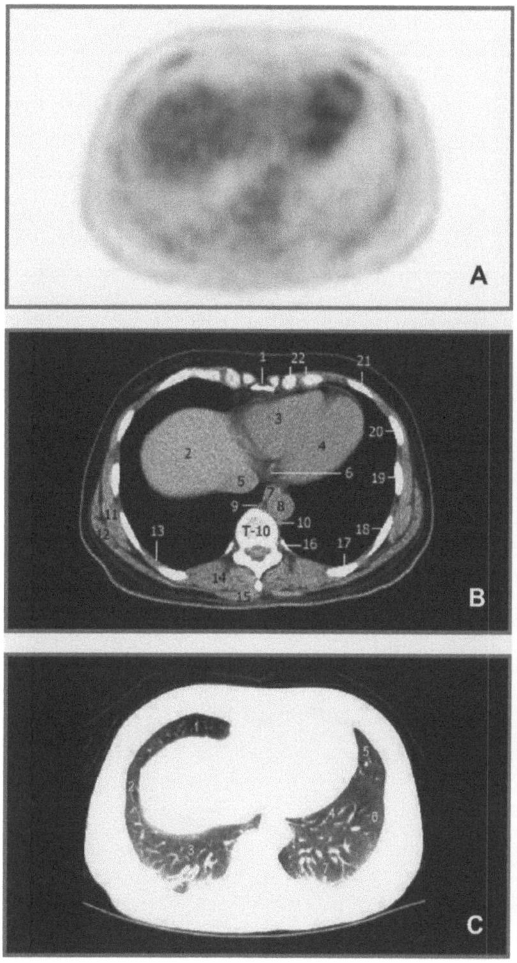

Picture 40

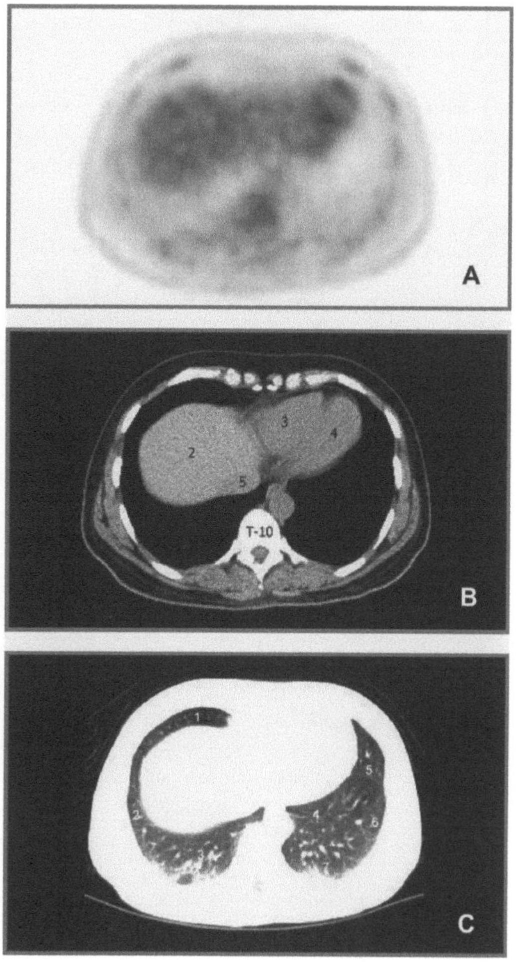

Keys

1. Sternum, xiphoid process
2. Liver
3. Right ventricle
4. Left ventricle
5. Inferior caval vein
6. Coronary sinus
7. Oesophagus
8. Thoracic aorta
9. Azygos vein
10. Hemiazygos vein
11. Serratus anterior
12. Latissimus dorsi
13. Intercostal muscles
14. Erector spinae
15. Trapezius
16. 10th rib
17. 9th rib
18. 8th rib
19. 7th rib
20. 6th rib
21. 5th rib
22. Osteochondral junction

Lung parenchymal window

1. Anterior basal segment, right lung inferior lobe
2. Lateral basal segment, right lung inferior lobe
3. Posterior basal segment, right lung inferior lobe
4. Medial basal segment, left lung inferior lobe
5. Anterior basal segment, left lung inferior lobe
6. Lateral basal segment, left lung inferior lobe
7. Posterior basal segment, left lung inferior lobe

Picture 41

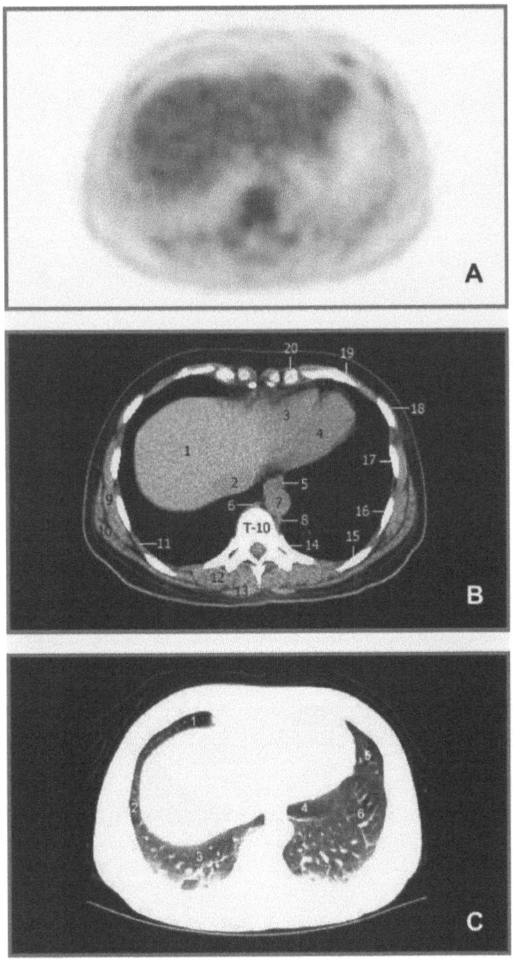

Picture 42

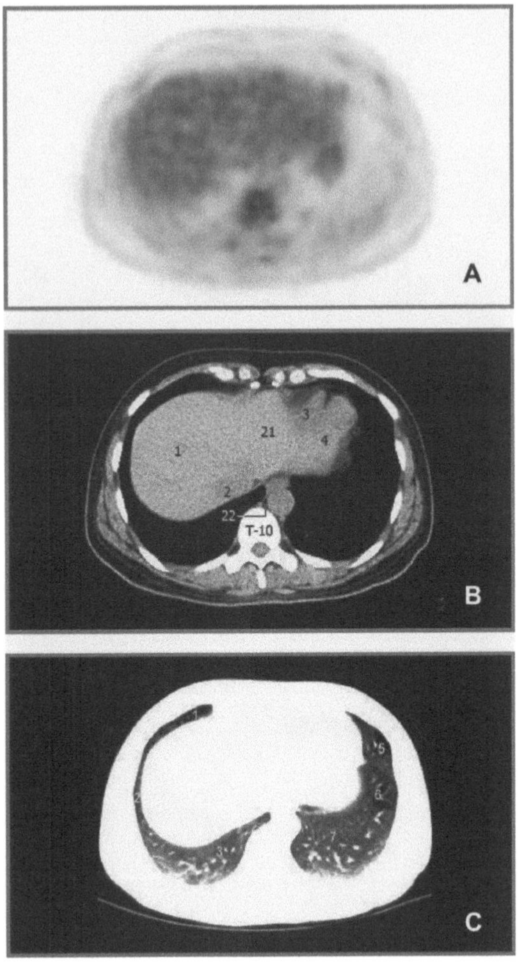

Keys

1. Right lobe of liver
2. Inferior caval vein
3. Right ventricle
4. Left ventricle
5. Oesophagus
6. Azygos vein
7. Thoracic aorta
8. Hemiazygos vein
9. Serratus anterior
10. Latissimus dorsi
11. Intercostal muscles
12. Erector spinae
13. Trapezius
14. 10th rib
15. 9th rib
16. 8th rib
17. 7th rib
18. 6th rib
19. 5th rib
20. Osteochondral junction
21. Left lobe of liver
22. Thoracic duct

Lung parenchymal window

1. Anterior basal segment, right lung inferior lobe
2. Lateral basal segment, right lung inferior lobe
3. Posterior basal segment, right lung inferior lobe
4. Medial basal segment, left lung inferior lobe
5. Anterior basal segment, left lung inferior lobe
6. Lateral basal segment, left lung inferior lobe
7. Posterior basal segment, left lung inferior lobe

Picture 43

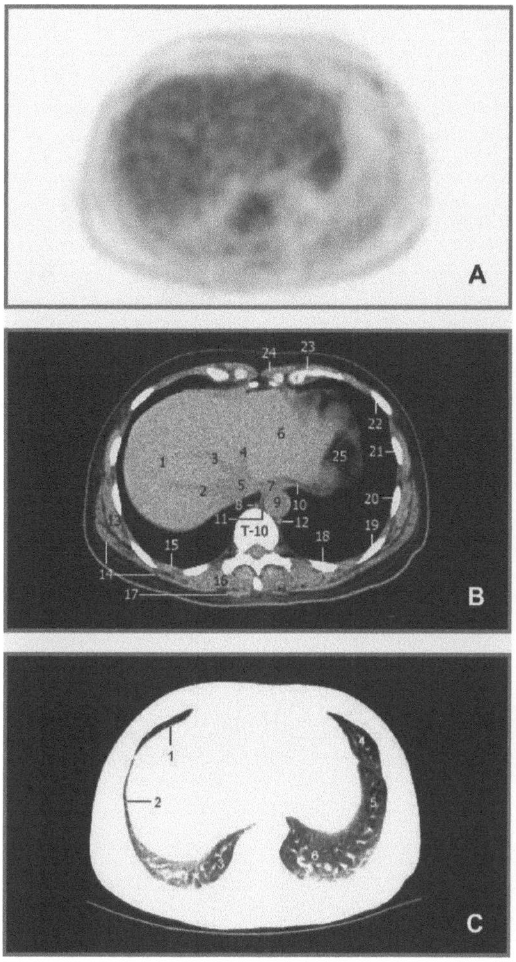

Picture 44

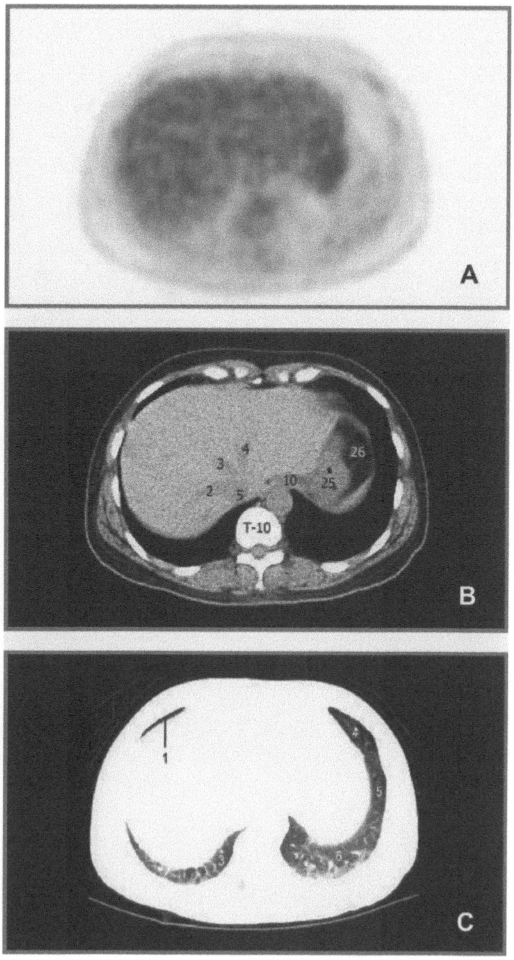

Keys

1. Right lobe of liver
2. Right hepatic vein
3. Intermediate hepatic vein
4. Left hepatic vein
5. Inferior caval vein
6. Left lobe of liver
7. Oesophagus
8. Azygos vein
9. Thoracic aorta
10. Gastroesophageal junction
11. Thoracic duct
12. Hemiazygos vein
13. Serratus anterior
14. Latissimus dorsi
15. Intercostal muscles
16. Erector spinae
17. Trapezius
18. 10th rib
19. 9th rib
20. 8th rib
21. 7th rib
22. 6th rib
23. Osteochondral junction
24. Rectus abdominis
25. Stomach, cardia
26. Fundus of stomach

Lung parenchymal window

1. Anterior basal segment, right lung inferior lobe
2. Lateral basal segment, right lung inferior lobe
3. Posterior basal segment, right lung inferior lobe
4. Anterior basal segment, left lung inferior lobe
5. Lateral basal segment, left lung inferior lobe
6. Posterior basal segment, left lung inferior lobe

Picture 45

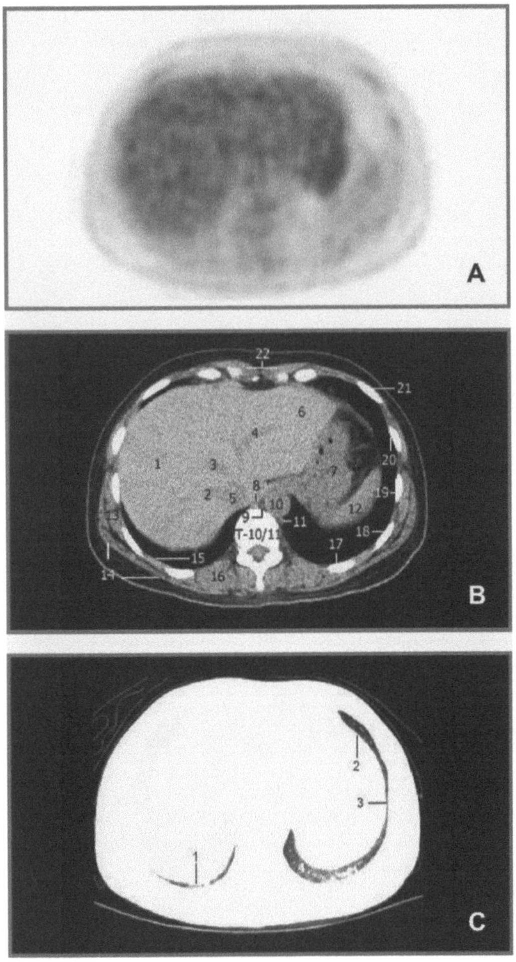

Picture 46

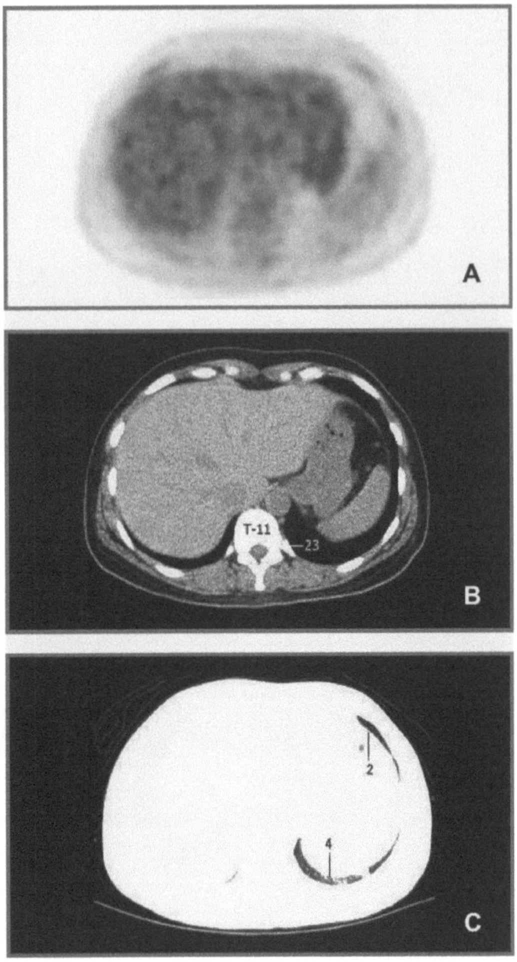

Keys

1. Right lobe of liver
2. Right hepatic vein
3. Intermediate hepatic vein
4. Left hepatic vein
5. Inferior caval vein
6. Left lobe of liver
7. Body of stomach
8. Azygos vein
9. Thoracic duct
10. Thoracic aorta
11. Hemiazygos vein
12. Spleen
13. Serratus anterior
14. Latissimus dorsi
15. Intercostal muscles
16. Erector spinae
17. 10th rib
18. 9th rib
19. 8th rib
20. 7th rib
21. 6th rib
22. Rectus abdominis
23. 11th rib

Lung parenchymal window

1. Posterior basal segment, left lung inferior lobe
2. Anterior basal segment, left lung inferior lobe
3. Lateral basal segment, left lung inferior lobe
4. Posterior basal segment, left lung inferior lobe

Chapter 3
Abdomen

M.T. Kitapçı, *Atlas of Sectional Radiological Anatomy for PET/CT*,
DOI 10.1007/978-1-4614-1527-5_3, © Springer Science+Business Media New York 2012

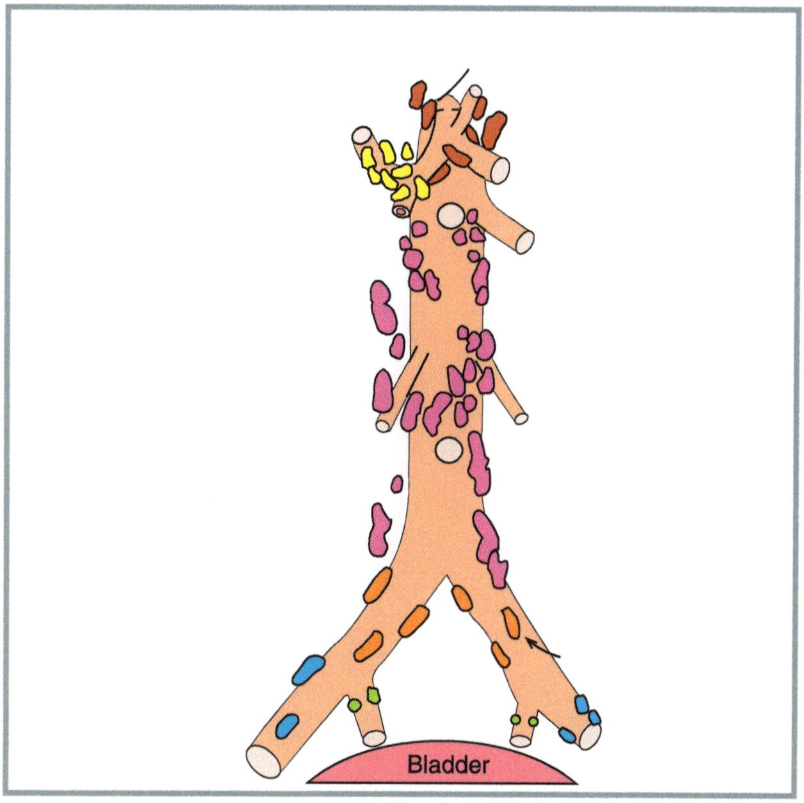

ABDOMEN

Lymph Nodes

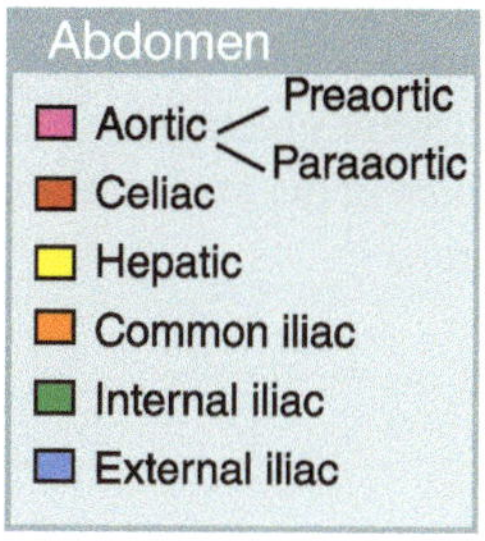

Adapted and modified from Moore KL, et al.

* *Moore KL, Dalley AF. II. Clinically Oriented Anatomy. 4th ed. Philadelphia: Lippincott Williams & Wilkins, 1999.*

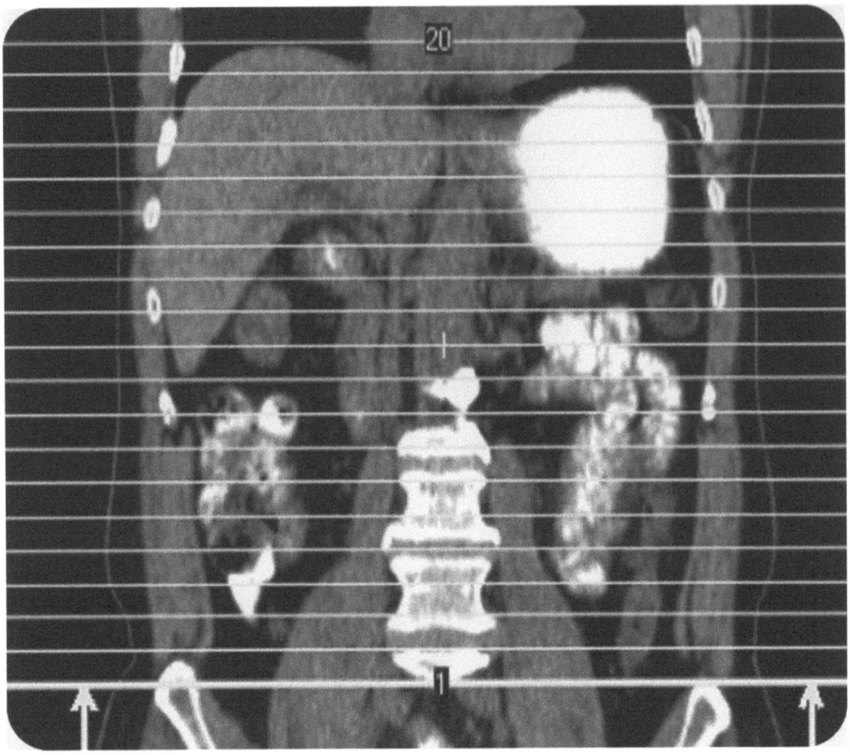

Consecutive sections were obtained with 3-mm slice thickness and without intravenous contrast. Positron Emission Tomography (PET) scintigraphic and Computed Tomography (CT) images obtained from the same level were given side to side for comparison. All anatomic structures in an image were numbered and given in the explanation section at the bottom of the page. Vertebral levels were marked on each vertebra.

Picture 1

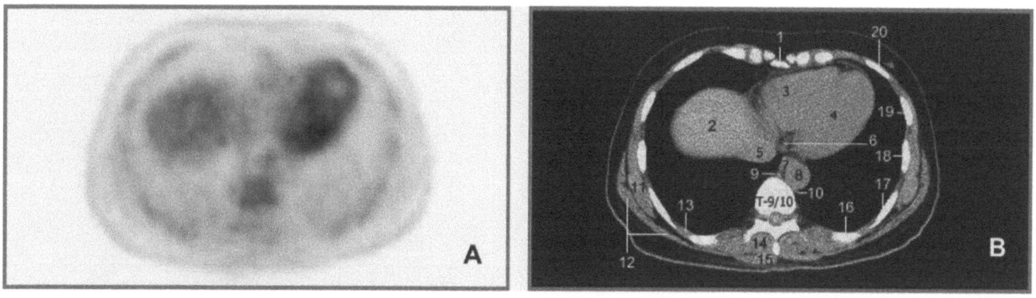

Picture 2

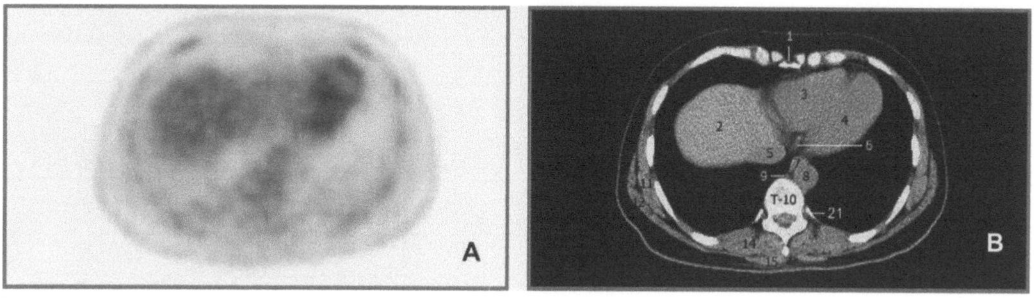

Picture 3

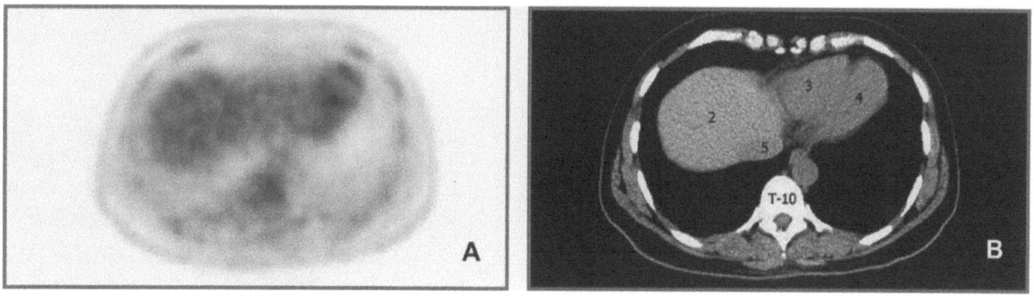

Keys

1. Sternum, xiphoid process
2. Liver
3. Right ventricle
4. Left ventricle
5. Inferior caval vein
6. Coronary sinus
7. Oesophagus
8. Thoracic aorta
9. Azygos vein
10. Hemiazygos vein
11. Serratus anterior
12. Latissimus dorsi
13. Intercostal muscles
14. Erector spinae
15. Trapezius
16. 9th rib
17. 8th rib
18. 7th rib
19. 6th rib
20. 5th rib
21. 10th rib

Picture 4

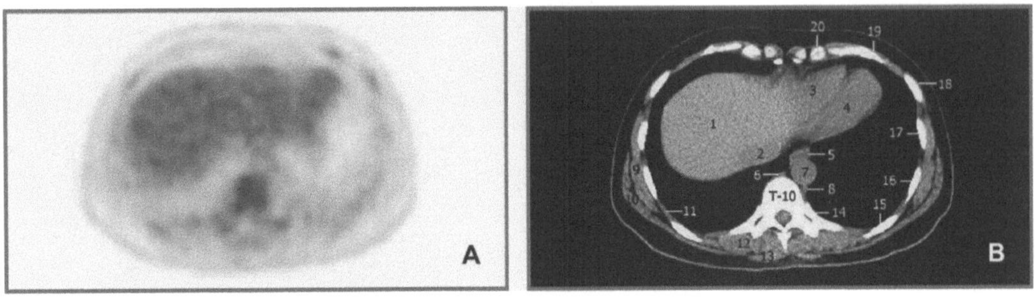

Picture 5

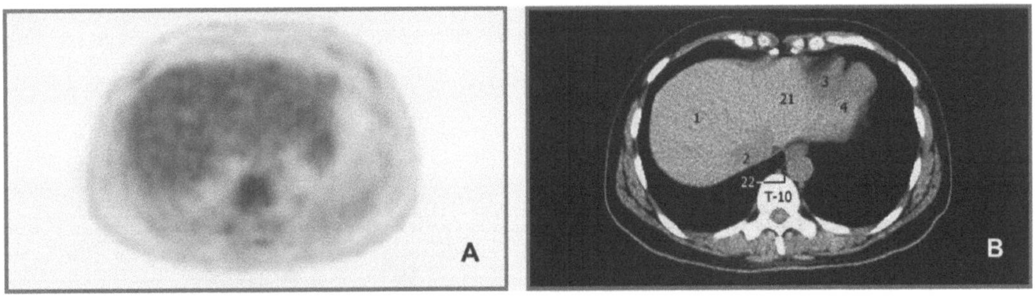

Picture 6

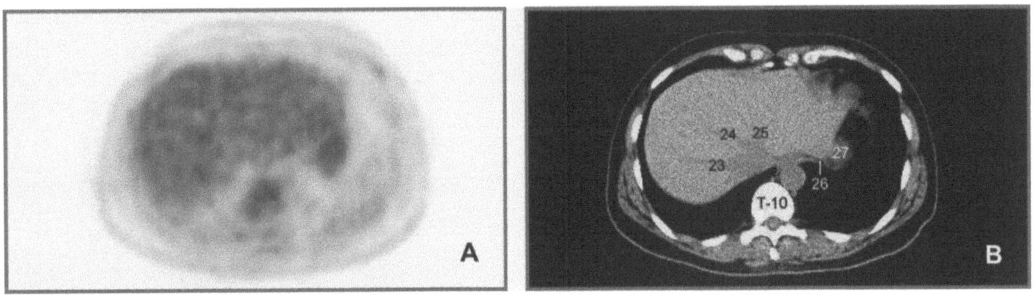

Keys

1. Right lobe of liver
2. Inferior caval vein
3. Right ventricle
4. Left ventricle
5. Oesophagus
6. Azygos vein
7. Thoracic aorta
8. Hemiazygos vein
9. Serratus anterior
10. Latissimus dorsi
11. Intercostal muscles
12. Erector spinae
13. Trapezius
14. 10th rib
15. 9th rib
16. 8th rib
17. 7th rib
18. 6th rib
19. 5th rib
20. Costochondral joint
21. Left lobe of liver
22. Thoracic duct
23. Right hepatic vein
24. Intermediate hepatic vein
25. Left hepatic vein
26. Gastro-oesophageal junction
27. Cardia of stomach

Picture 7

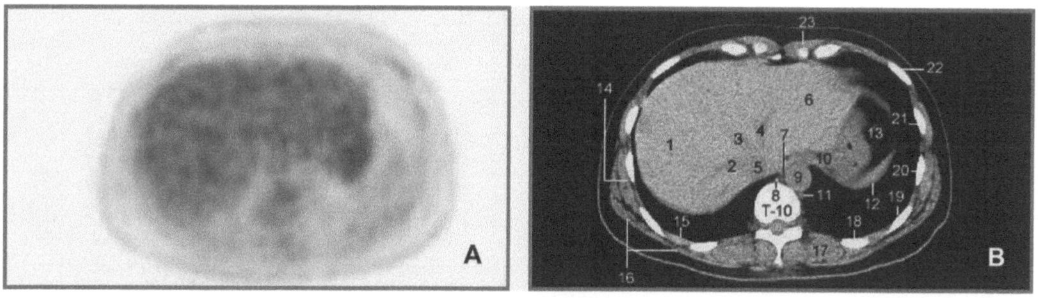

Picture 8

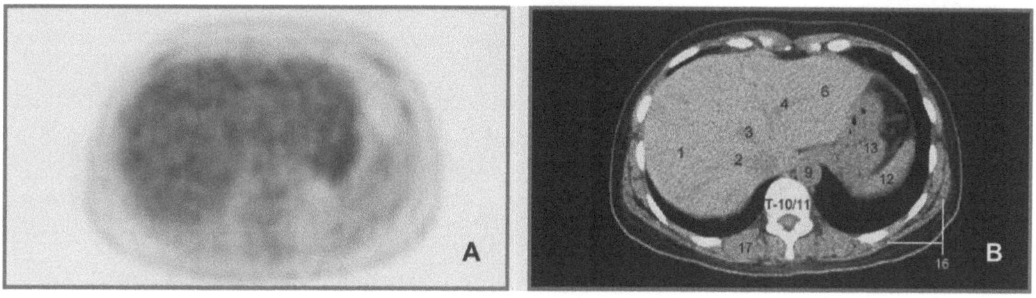

Picture 9

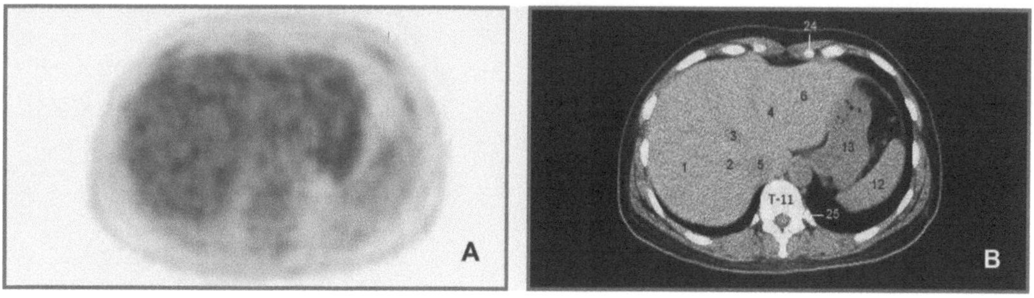

Keys

1. Right lobe of liver
2. Right hepatic vein
3. Intermediate hepatic vein
4. Left hepatic vein
5. Inferior caval vein
6. Left lobe of liver
7. Thoracic duct
8. Azygos vein
9. Thoracic aorta
10. Cardia of stomach
11. Hemiazygos vein
12. Spleen
13. Body of stomach
14. Serratus anterior
15. Intercostal muscles
16. Latissimus dorsi
17. Erector spinae
18. 10th rib
19. 9th rib
20. 8th rib
21. 7th rib
22. 6th rib
23. Rectus abdominis
24. Costochondral joint
25. 11th rib

Picture 10

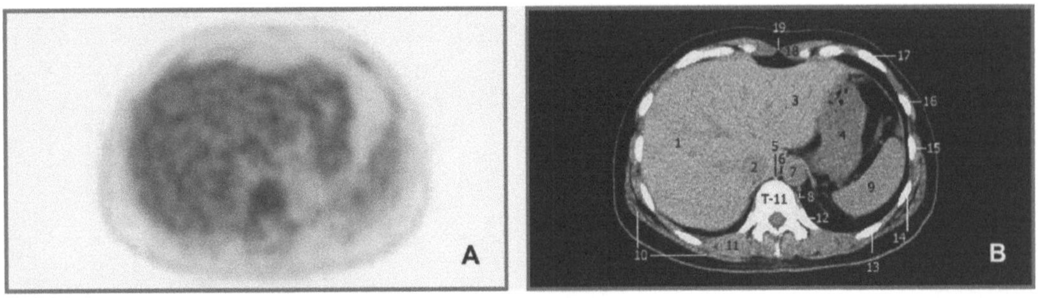

Picture 11

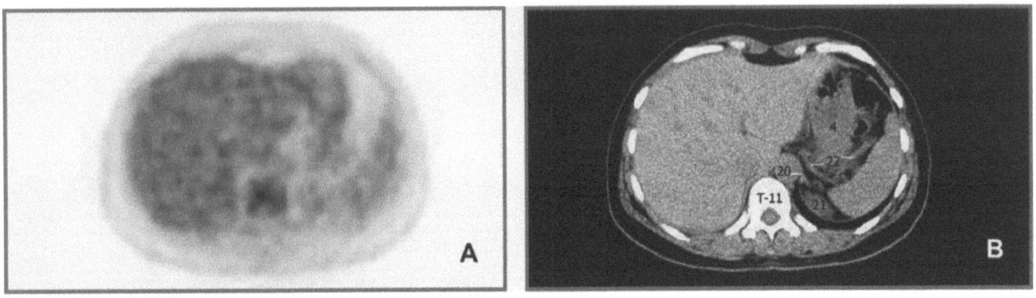

Picture 12

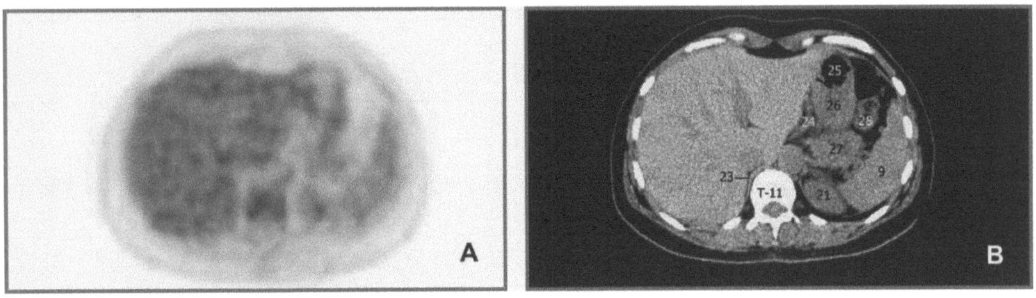

Keys

1. Right lobe of liver
2. Inferior caval vein
3. Left lobe of liver
4. Body of stomach
5. Azygos vein
6. Thoracic duct
7. Thoracic aorta
8. Hemiazygos vein
9. Spleen
10. Latissimus dorsi
11. Erector spinae
12. 11th rib
13. 10th rib
14. 9th rib
15. 8th rib
16. 7th rib
17. 6th rib
18. Rectus abdominis
19. Linea alba
20. Left adrenal gland
21. Upper pole of left kidney
22. Splenic artery
23. Right crus of diaphragm
24. Left gastric artery
25. Transverse colon
26. Pyloric antrum of stomach
27. Body of pancreas
28. Left colic flexure

Picture 13

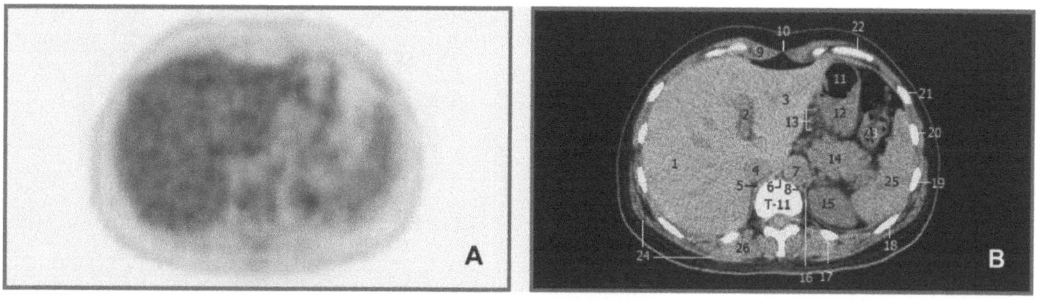

Picture 14

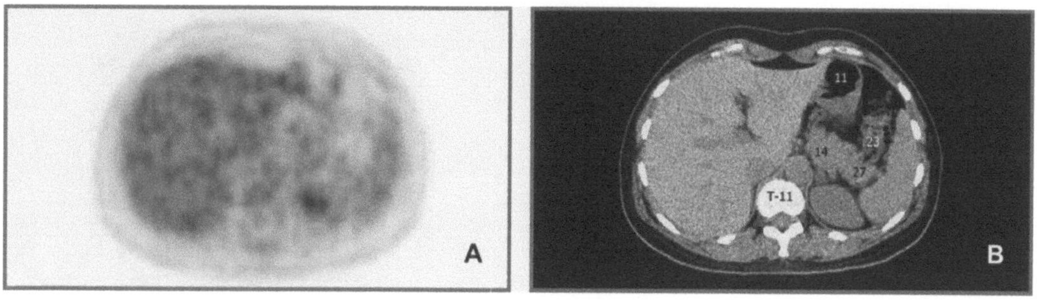

Picture 15

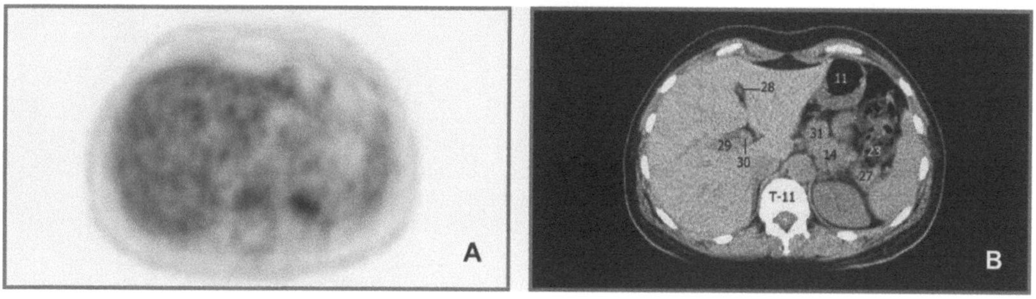

Keys

1. Right lobe of liver
2. Left branch of portal vein
3. Left lobe of liver
4. Inferior caval vein
5. Right crus of diaphragm
6. Thoracic duct
7. Thoracic aorta
8. Hemiazygos vein
9. Rectus abdominis
10. Linea alba
11. Transverse colon
12. Pyloric antrum of stomach
13. Left gastric artery
14. Body of pancreas
15. Left kidney
16. Left crus of diaphragm
17. 11th rib
18. 10th rib
19. 9th rib
20. 8th rib
21. 7th rib
22. 6th rib
23. Left colic flexure
24. Latissimus dorsi
25. Spleen
26. Erector spinae
27. Tail of pancreas
28. Round ligament of liver
29. Right branch of portal vein
30. Portal vein

Picture 16

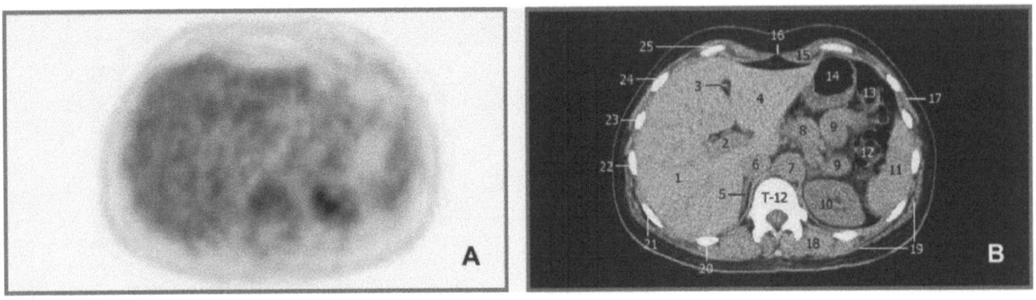

Picture 17

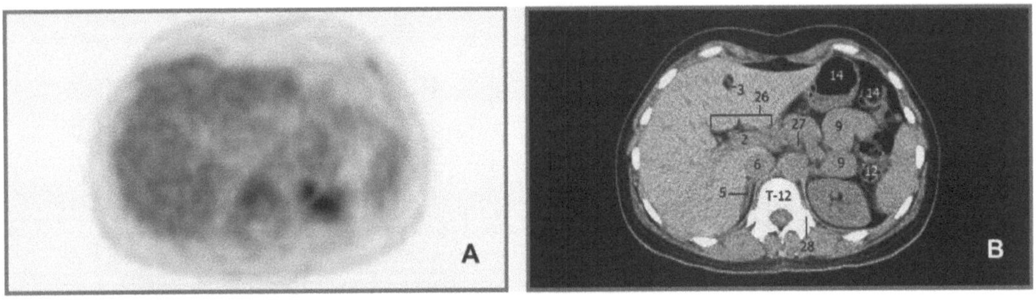

Picture 18

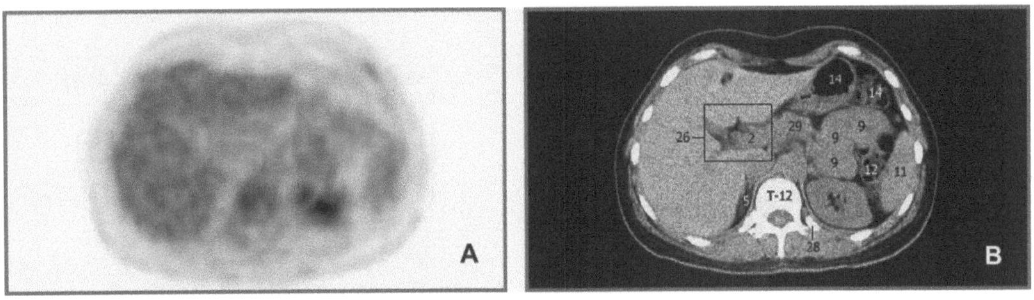

Keys

1. Right lobe of liver
2. Portal vein
3. Round ligament of liver
4. Left lobe of liver
5. Right adrenal gland
6. Inferior caval vein
7. Abdominal aorta
8. Head of pancreas
9. Jejunum
10. Left kidney
11. Spleen
12. Descending colon
13. Left colic flexure
14. Transverse colon
15. Rectus abdominis
16. Linea alba
17. Obliquus externus abdominis
18. Erector spinae
19. Latissimus dorsi
20. 11th rib
21. 10th rib
22. 9th rib
23. 8th rib
24. 7th rib
25. 6th rib
26. Porta hepatis
27. Celiac trunk
28. 12th rib
29. Duodenum

Picture 19

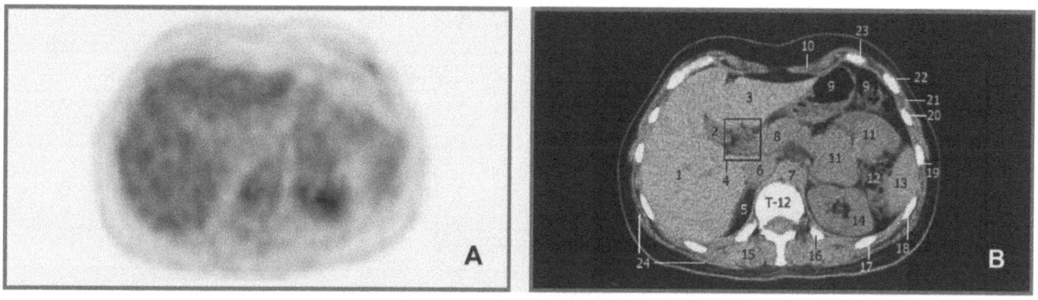

Picture 20

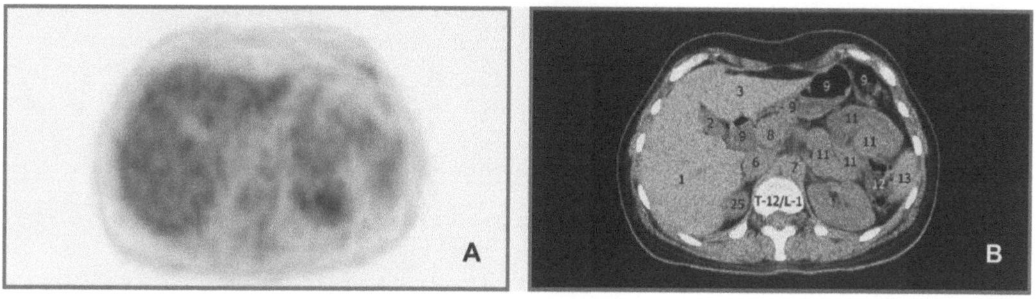

Picture 21

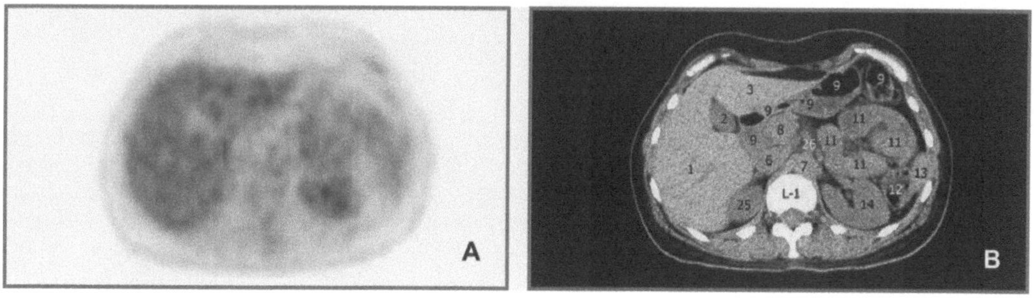

Keys

1. Right lobe of liver
2. Gall bladder
3. Left lobe of liver
4. Porta hepatis
5. Right adrenal gland region
6. Inferior caval vein
7. Abdominal aorta
8. Duodenum
9. Transverse colon
10. Rectus abdominis
11. Jejunum
12. Descending colon
13. Spleen
14. Left kidney
15. Erector spinae
16. 12th rib
17. 11th rib
18. 10th rib
19. 9th rib
20. 8th rib
21. Obliquus externus abdominis
22. 7th rib
23. 6th rib
24. Latissimus dorsi
25. Upper pole of right kidney
26. Superior mesenteric artery

Picture 22

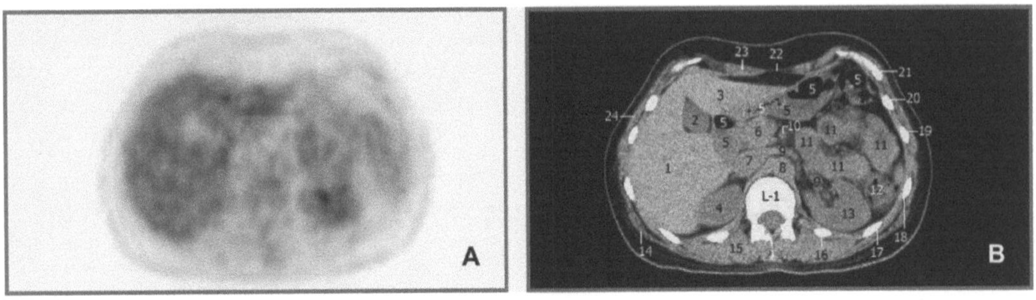

Picture 23

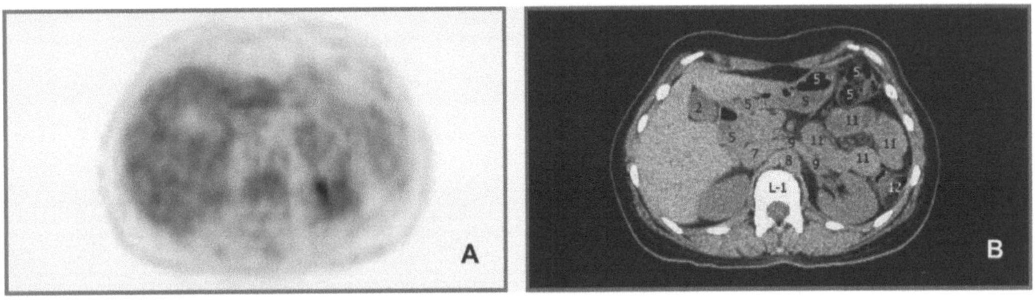

Picture 24

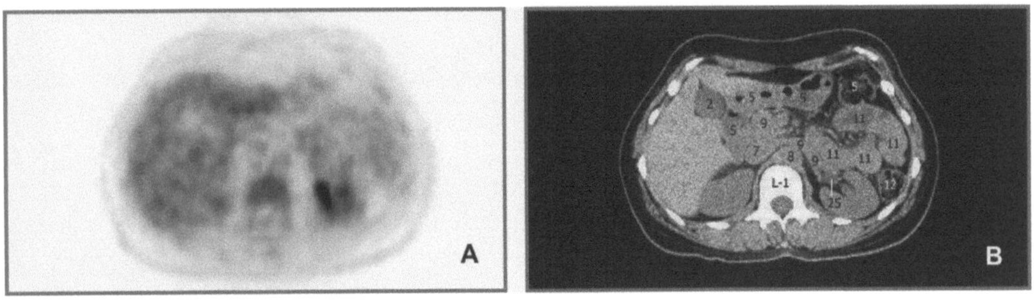

Keys

1. Right lobe of liver
2. Gall bladder
3. Left lobe of liver
4. Upper pole of right kidney
5. Transverse colon
6. Duodenum
7. Inferior caval vein
8. Abdominal aorta
9. Left renal vein
10. Superior mesenteric artery
11. Jejunum
12. Descending colon
13. Left kidney
14. Latissimus dorsi
15. Erector spinae
16. 12th rib
17. 11th rib
18. 10th rib
19. 9th rib
20. 8th rib
21. 7th rib
22. Linea alba
23. Rectus abdominis
24. Obliquus externus abdominis
25. Left renal pelvis

Picture 25

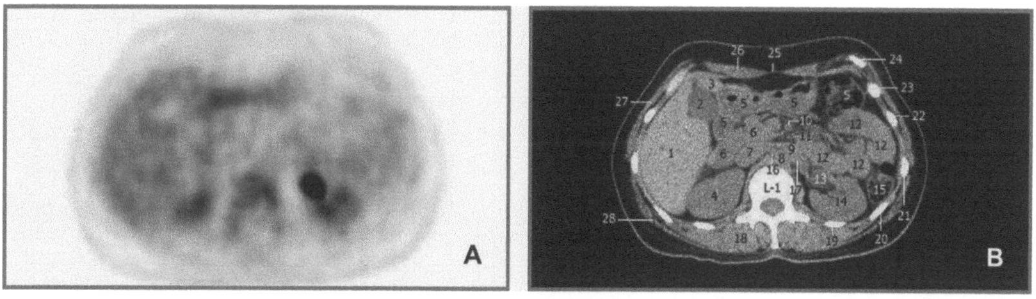

Picture 26

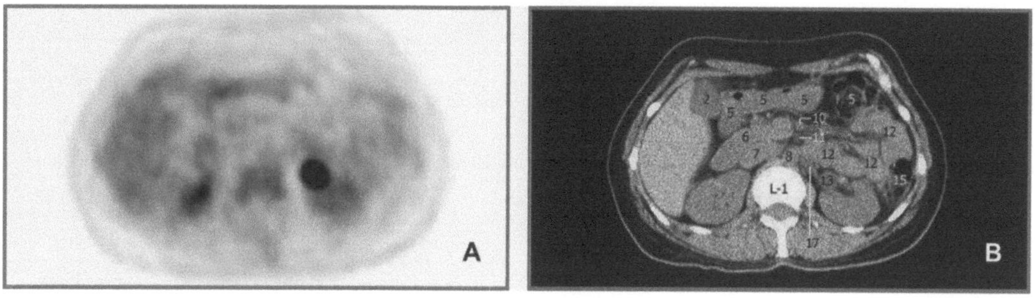

Picture 27

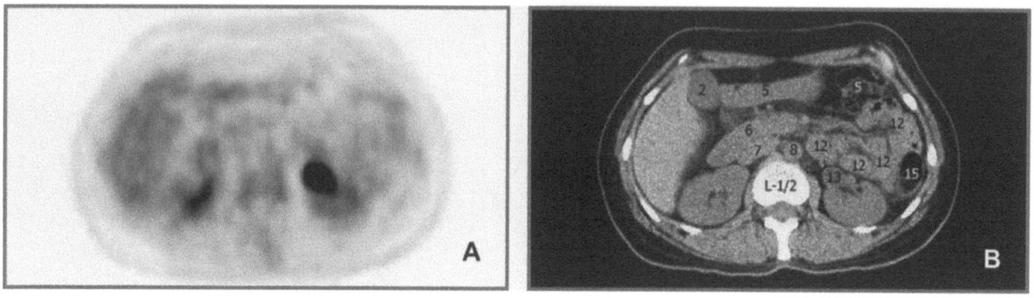

Keys

1. Right lobe of liver
2. Gall bladder
3. Left lobe of liver
4. Right kidney
5. Transverse colon
6. Duodenum
7. Inferior caval vein
8. Abdominal aorta
9. Left renal vein
10. Superior mesenteric artery
11. Superior mesenteric vein
12. Jejunum
13. Left renal pelvis
14. Left kidney
15. Descending colon
16. Cisterna chyli
17. Left renal artery
18. Erector spinae
19. 12th rib
20. 11th rib
21. 10th rib
22. 9th rib
23. 8th rib
24. 7th rib
25. Linea alba
26. Rectus abdominis
27. Obliquus externus abdominis
28. Latissimus dorsi

Picture 25

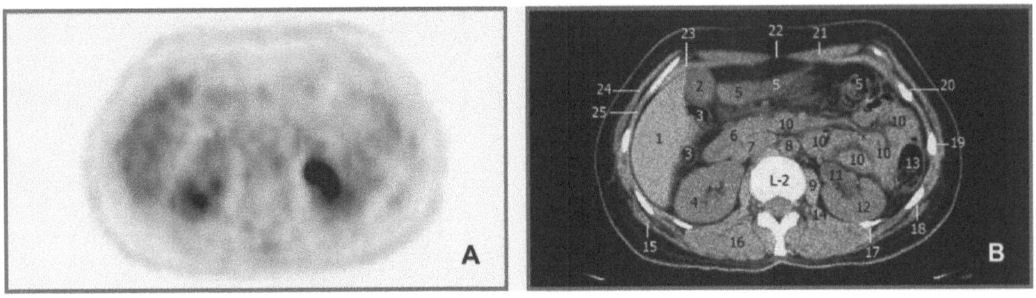

Picture 26

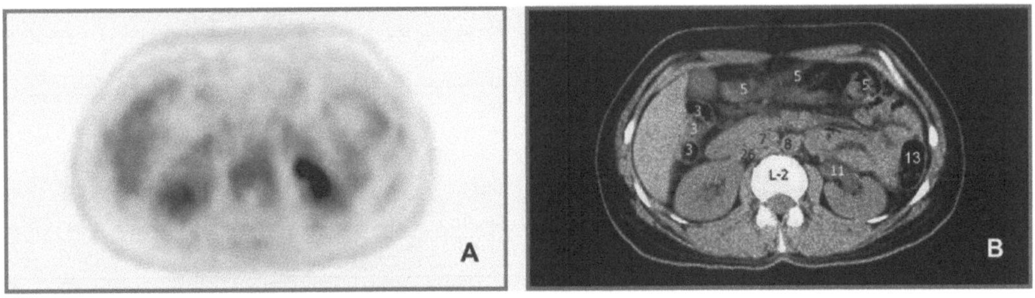

Picture 27

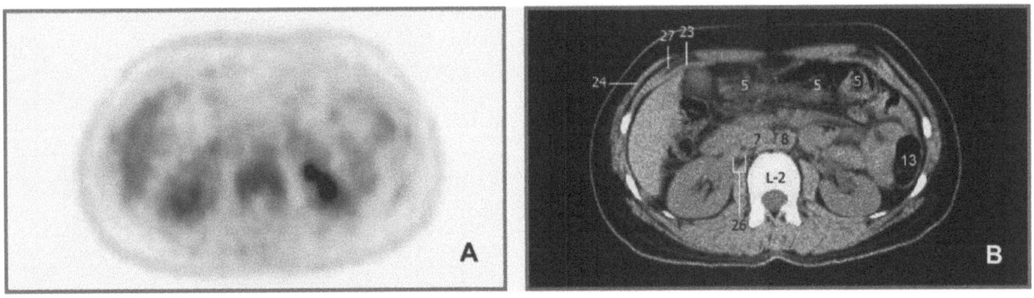

Keys

1. Right lobe of liver
2. Gall bladder
3. Right colic flexure
4. Right kidney
5. Transverse colon
6. Duodenum
7. Inferior caval vein
8. Abdominal aorta
9. Psoas major
10. Jejunum
11. Left renal pelvis
12. Left kidney
13. Descending colon
14. Quadratus lumborum
15. Latissimus dorsi
16. Erector spinae
17. 12th rib
18. 11th rib
19. 10th rib
20. 9th rib
21. Rectus abdominis
22. Linea alba
23. Transversus abdominis
24. Obliquus externus abdominis
25. Intercostal muscles
26. Right renal artery
27. Obliquus internus abdominis

Picture 28

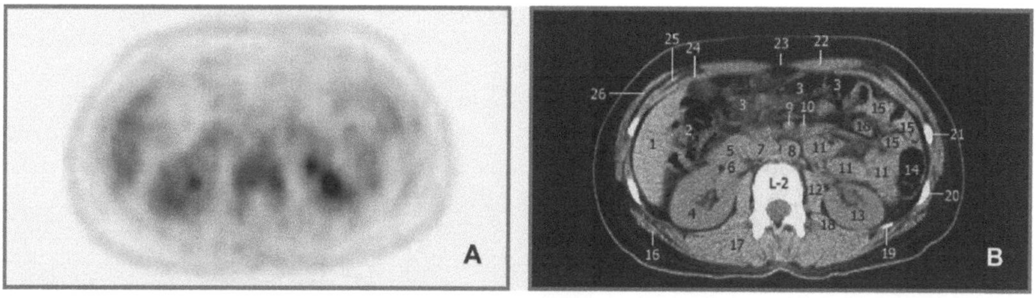

Picture 29

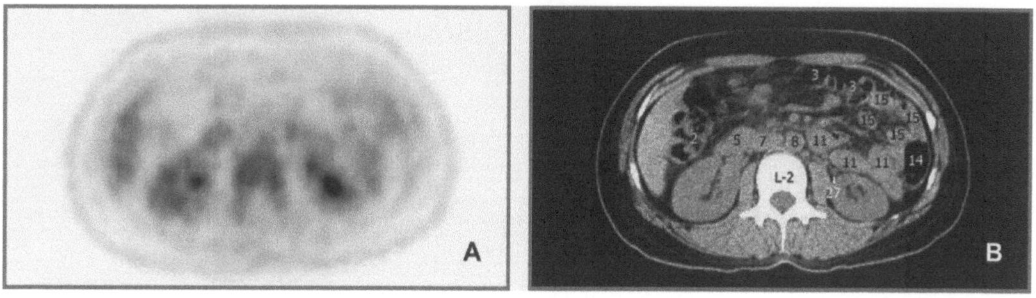

Picture 30

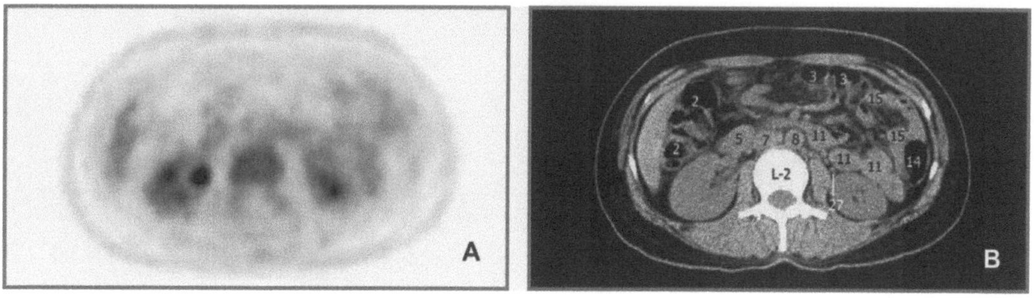

Keys

1. Right lobe of liver
2. Right colic flexure
3. Transverse colon
4. Right kidney
5. Duodenum
6. Right renal vein
7. Inferior caval vein
8. Abdominal aorta
9. Superior mesenteric vein
10. Superior mesenteric artery
11. Jejunum
12. Psoas major
13. Left kidney
14. Descending colon
15. Ileum
16. Latissimus dorsi
17. Erector spinae
18. Quadratus lumborum
19. 12th rib
20. 11th rib
21. 10th rib
22. Rectus abdominis
23. Linea alba
24. Transversus abdominis
25. Obliquus internus abdominis
26. Obliquus externus abdominis
27. Left ureter

Picture 31

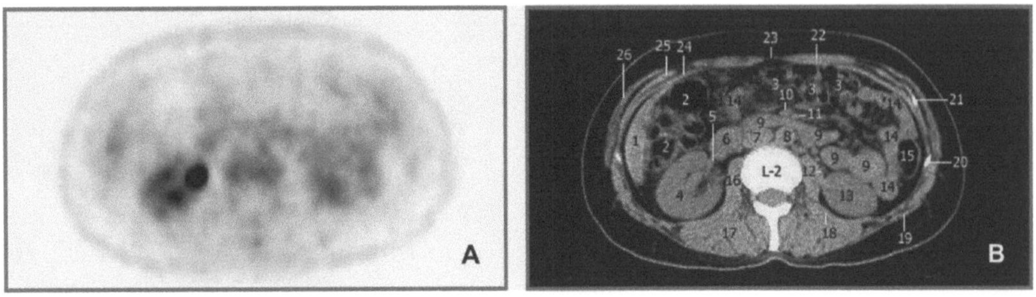

Picture 32

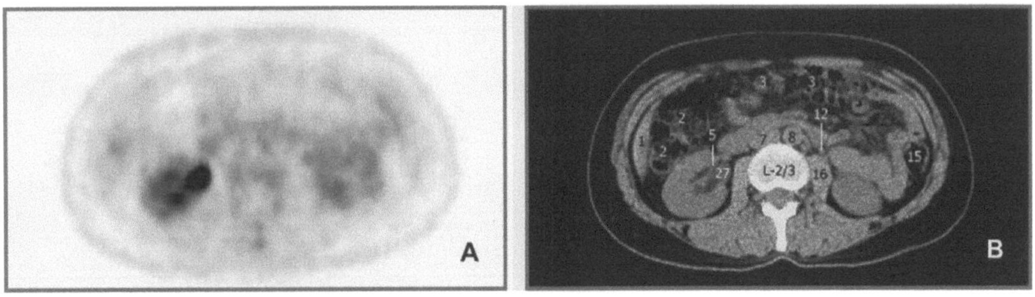

Picture 33

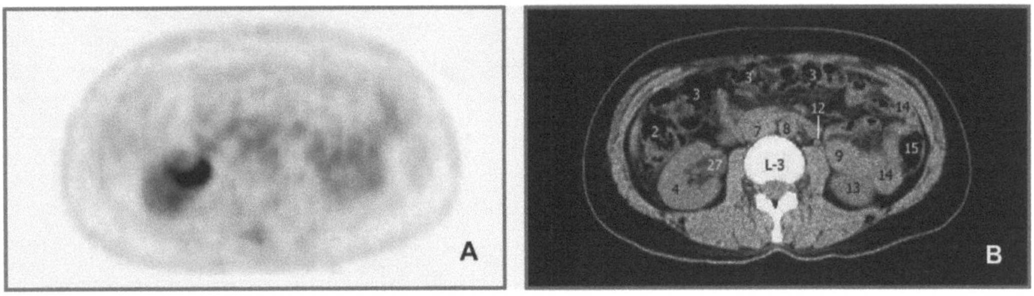

Keys

1. Right lobe of liver
2. Right colic flexure
3. Transverse colon
4. Right kidney
5. Right renal vein
6. Duodenum
7. Inferior caval vein
8. Abdominal aorta
9. Jejunum
10. Superior mesenteric vein
11. Superior mesenteric artery
12. Left ureter
13. Left kidney
14. Ileum
15. Descending colon
16. Psoas major
17. Erector spinae
18. Quadratus lumborum
19. Latissimus dorsi
20. 11th rib
21. 10th rib
22. Rectus abdominis
23. Linea alba
24. Transversus abdominis
25. Obliquus internus abdominis
26. Obliquus externus abdominis
27. Right renal pelvis

Picture 34

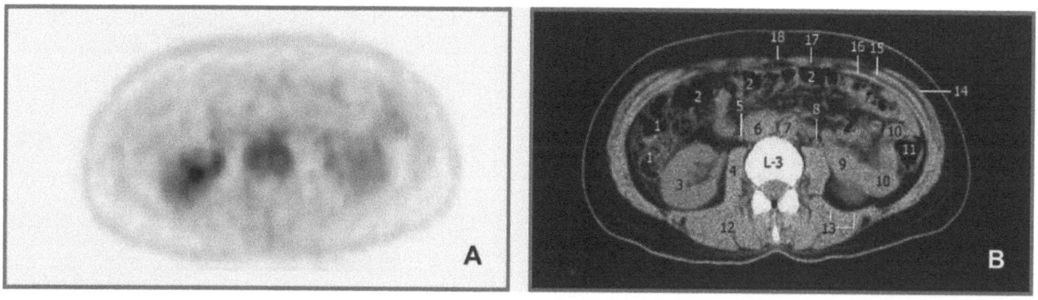

Picture 35

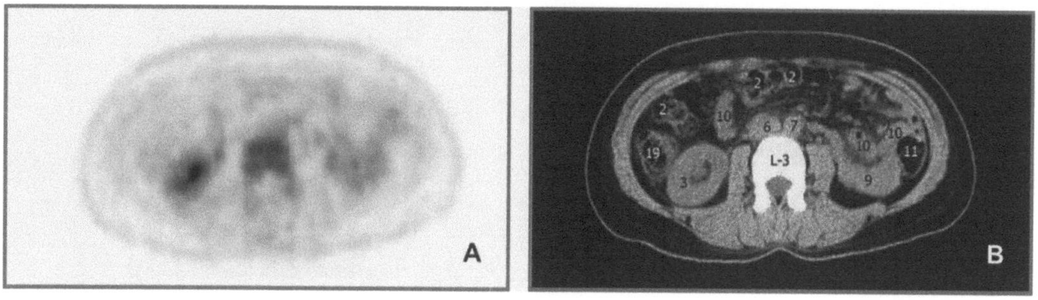

Picture 36

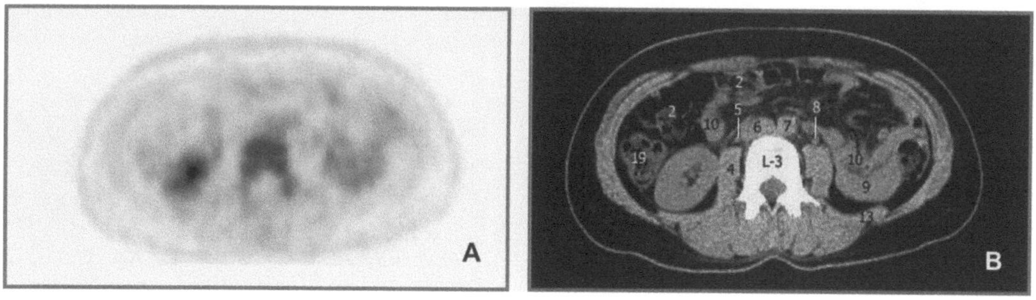

Keys

1. Right colic flexure
2. Transverse colon
3. Right kidney
4. Psoas major
5. Right ureter
6. Inferior caval vein
7. Abdominal aorta
8. Left ureter
9. Jejunum
10. Ileum
11. Descending colon
12. Erector spinae
13. Quadratus lumborum
14. Obliquus externus abdominis
15. Obliquus internus abdominis
16. Transversus abdominis
17. Rectus abdominis
18. Linea alba
19. Ascending colon

Picture 37

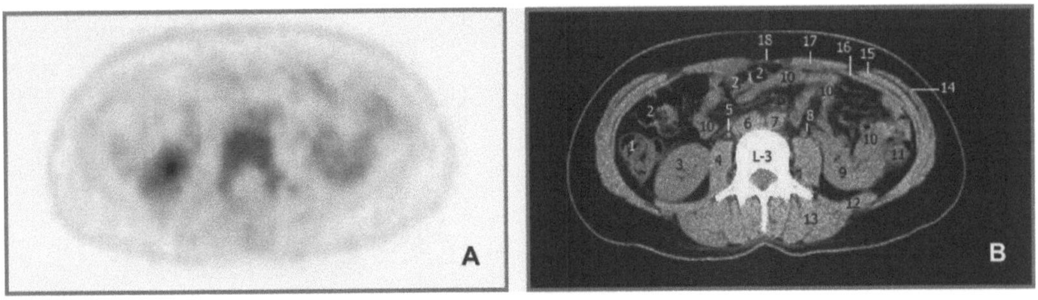

Picture 38

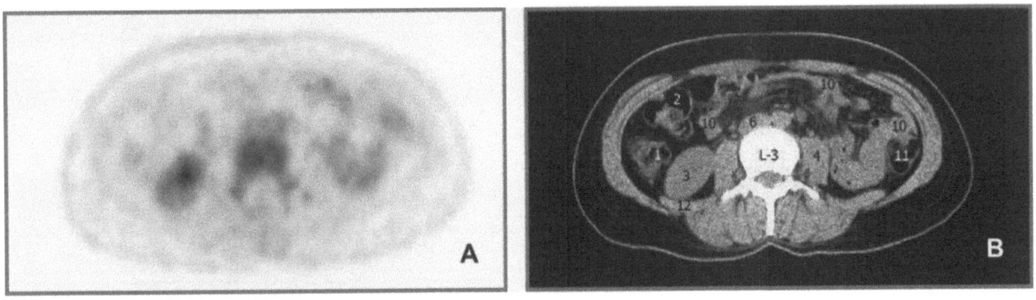

Picture 39

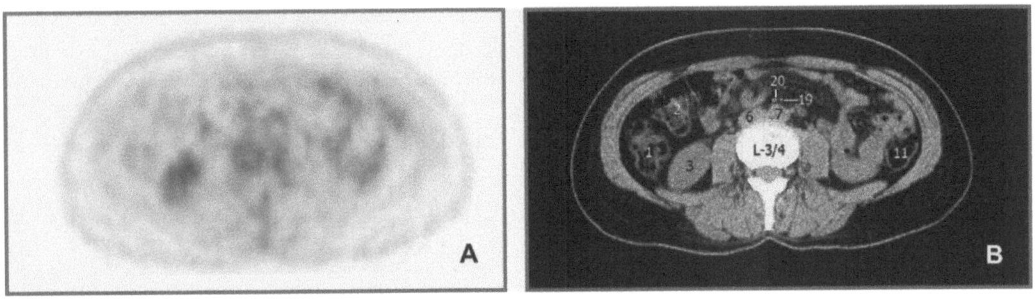

Keys

1. Ascending colon
2. Transverse colon
3. Right kidney
4. Psoas major
5. Right ureter
6. Inferior caval vein
7. Aortic bifurcation
8. Left ureter
9. Jejunum
10. Ileum
11. Descending colon
12. Quadratus lumborum
13. Erector spinae
14. Obliquus externus abdominis
15. Obliquus internus abdominis
16. Transversus abdominis
17. Rectus abdominis
18. Linea alba
19. Inferior mesenteric artery
20. Inferior mesenteric vein

Picture 40

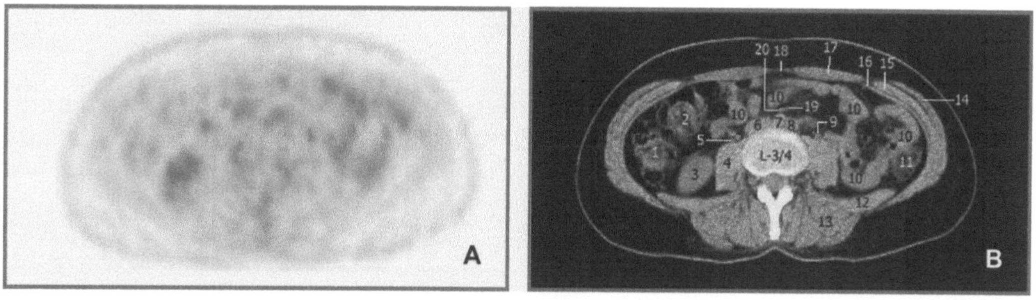

Picture 41

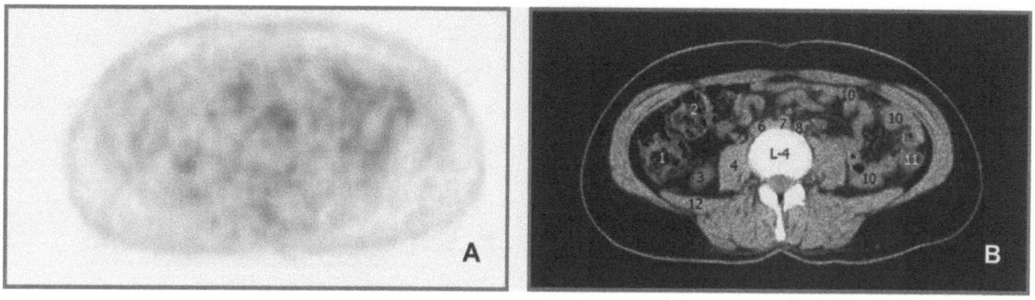

Picture 42

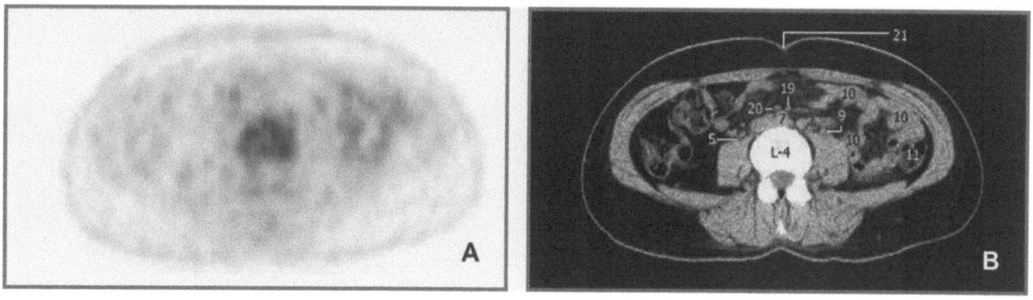

Keys

1. Ascending colon
2. Transverse colon
3. Lower pole of right kidney
4. Psoas major
5. Right ureter
6. Inferior caval vein
7. Right common iliac artery
8. Left common iliac artery
9. Left ureter
10. Ileum
11. Descending colon
12. Quadratus lumborum
13. Erector spinae
14. Obliquus externus abdominis
15. Obliquus internus abdominis
16. Transversus abdominis
17. Rectus abdominis
18. Linea alba
19. Inferior mesenteric artery
20. Inferior mesenteric vein
21. Umbilicus

Picture 43

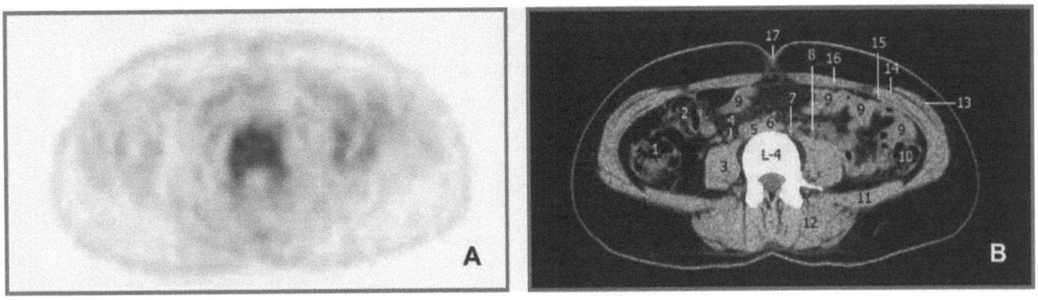

Picture 44

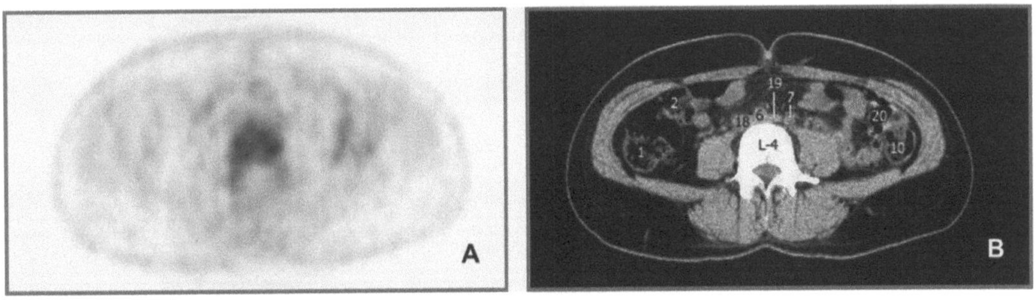

Picture 45

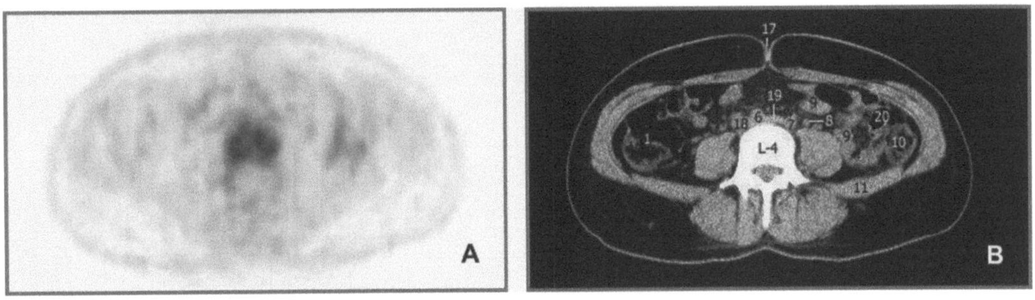

Keys

1. Ascending colon
2. Transverse colon
3. Psoas major
4. Right ureter
5. Inferior caval vein
6. Right common iliac artery
7. Left common iliac artery
8. Left ureter
9. Ileum
10. Descending colon
11. Quadratus lumborum
12. Erector spinae
13. Obliquus externus abdominis
14. Obliquus internus abdominis
15. Transversus abdominis
16. Rectus abdominis
17. Umbilicus
18. Right common iliac vein
19. Left common iliac vein
20. Sigmoid colon

Picture 46

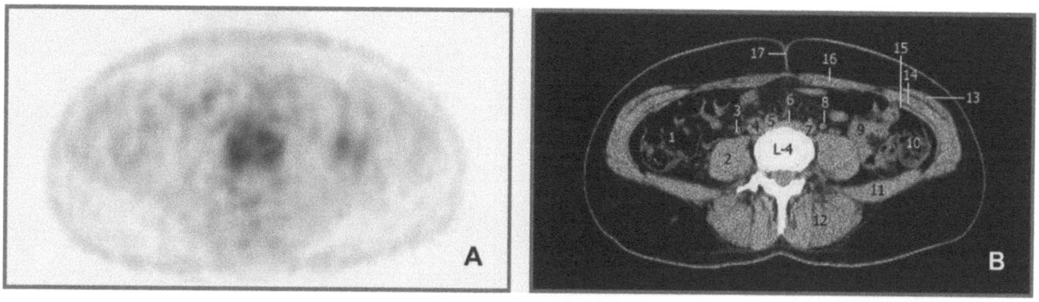

Picture 47

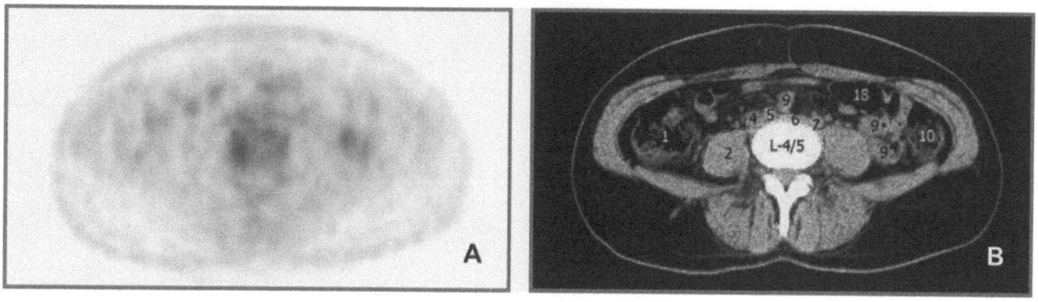

Picture 48

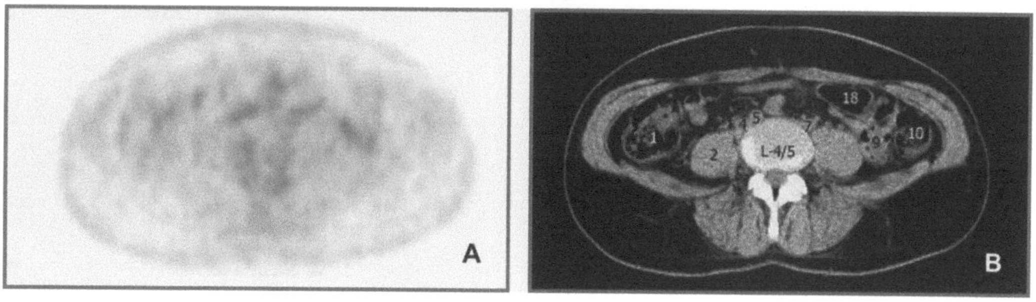

Keys

1. Ascending colon
2. Psoas major
3. Right ureter
4. Right common iliac vein
5. Right common iliac artery
6. Left common iliac vein
7. Left common iliac artery
8. Left ureter
9. Ileum
10. Descending colon
11. Quadratus lumborum
12. Erector spinae
13. Obliquus externus abdominis
14. Obliquus internus abdominis
15. Transversus abdominis
16. Rectus abdominis
17. Umbilicus
18. Sigmoid colon

Picture 49

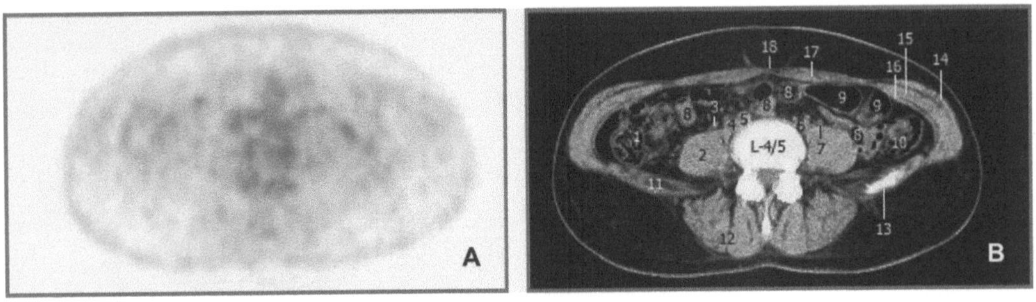

Picture 50

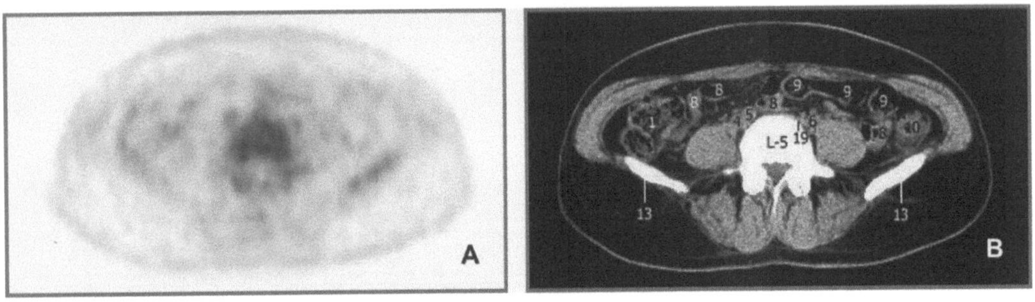

Picture 51

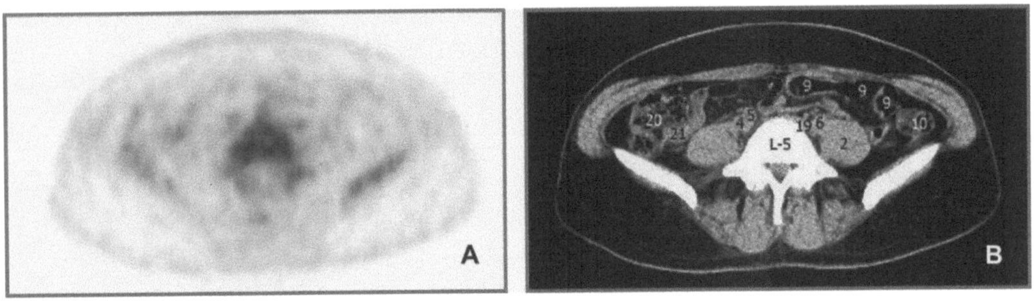

Keys

1. Ascending colon
2. Psoas major
3. Right ureter
4. Right common iliac vein
5. Right common iliac artery
6. Left common iliac artery
7. Left ureter
8. Ileum
9. Sigmoid colon
10. Descending colon
11. Quadratus lumborum
12. Erector spinae
13. Iliac crest
14. Obliquus externus abdominis
15. Obliquus internus abdominis
16. Transversus abdominis
17. Rectus abdominis
18. Linea alba
19. Left common iliac vein
20. Caecum
21. Terminal ileum

Picture 52

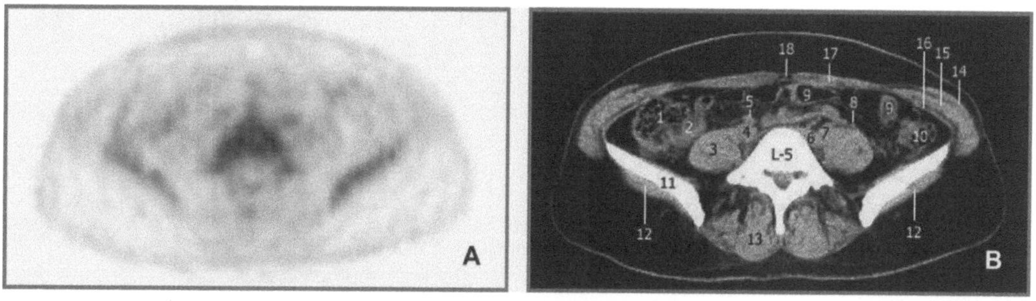

Picture 53

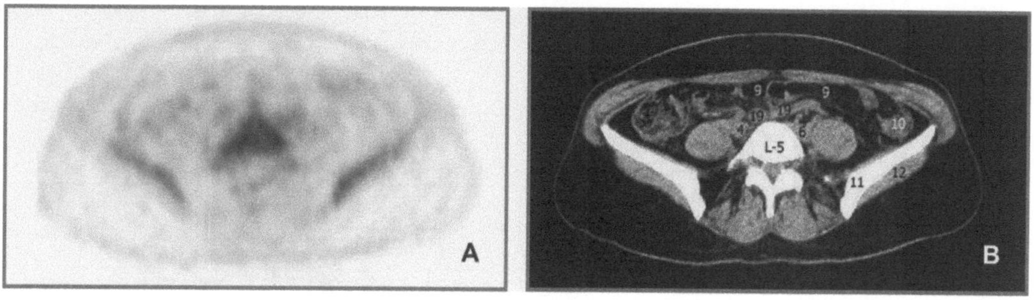

Picture 54

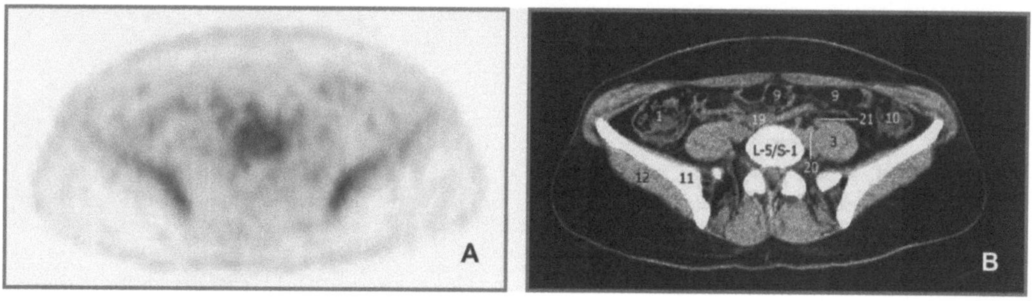

Keys

1. Caecum
2. Terminal ileum
3. Psoas major
4. Right common iliac vein
5. Right common iliac artery
6. Left common iliac vein
7. Left common iliac artery
8. Left ureter
9. Sigmoid colon
10. Descending colon
11. Iliac crest
12. Gluteus medius
13. Erector spinae
14. Obliquus externus abdominis
15. Obliquus internus abdominis
16. Transversus abdominis
17. Rectus abdominis
18. Linea alba
19. Ileum
20. Left internal iliac artery
21. Left external iliac artery

Picture 55

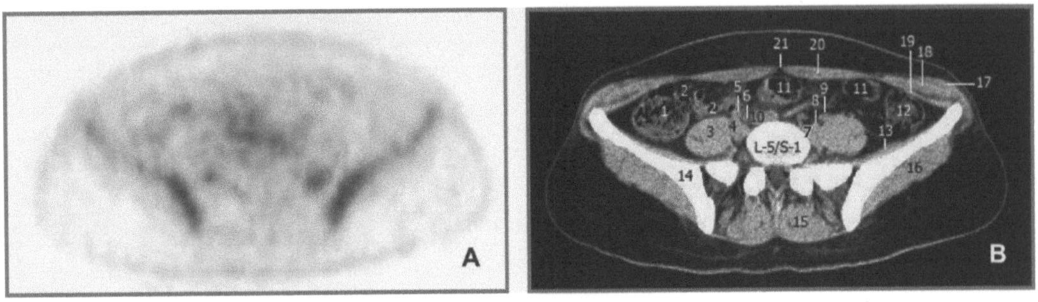

Picture 56

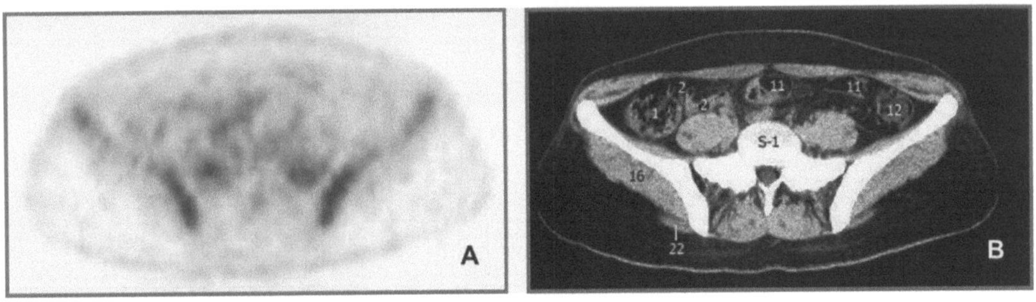

Picture 57

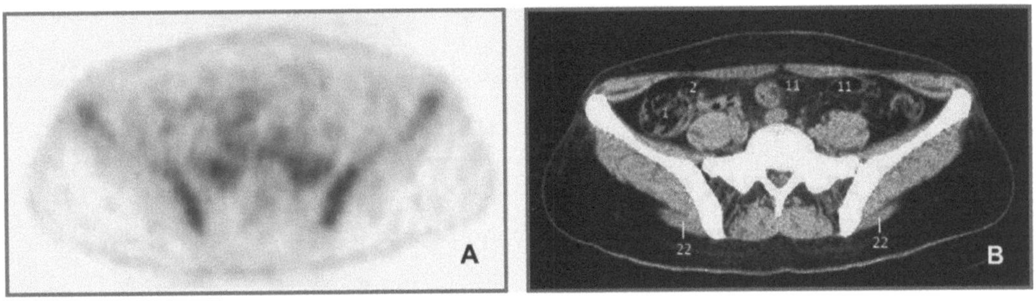

Keys

1. Caecum
2. Terminal ileum
3. Psoas major
4. Right common iliac vein
5. Right external iliac artery
6. Right internal iliac artery
7. Left common iliac vein
8. Left internal iliac artery
9. Left external iliac artery
10. Ileum
11. Sigmoid colon
12. Descending colon
13. Iliacus
14. Iliac crest
15. Erector spinae
16. Gluteus medius
17. Obliquus externus abdominis
18. Obliquus internus abdominis
19. Transversus abdominis
20. Rectus abdominis
21. Linea alba
22. Gluteus maximus

Picture 58

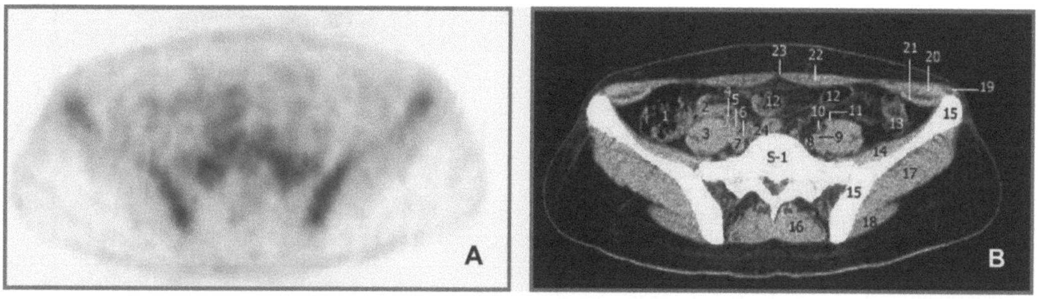

Picture 59

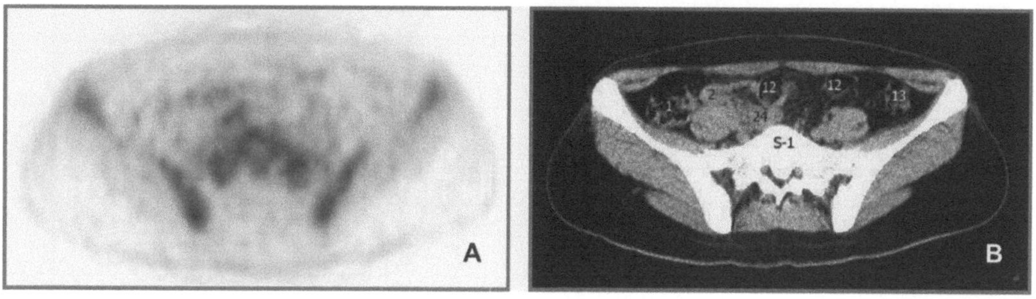

Picture 60

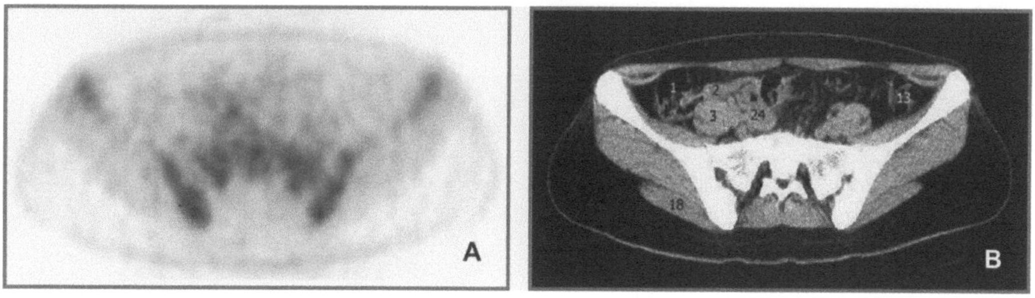

Keys

1. Caecum
2. Terminal ileum
3. Psoas major
4. Right external iliac artery
5. Right external iliac vein
6. Right internal iliac artery
7. Right internal iliac vein
8. Left internal iliac vein
9. Left internal iliac artery
10. Left external iliac vein
11. Left external iliac artery
12. Sigmoid colon
13. Descending colon
14. Iliacus
15. Iliac crest
16. Erector spinae
17. Gluteus medius
18. Gluteus maximus
19. Obliquus externus abdominis
20. Obliquus internus abdominis
21. Transversus abdominis
22. Rectus abdominis
23. Linea alba
24. Ileum

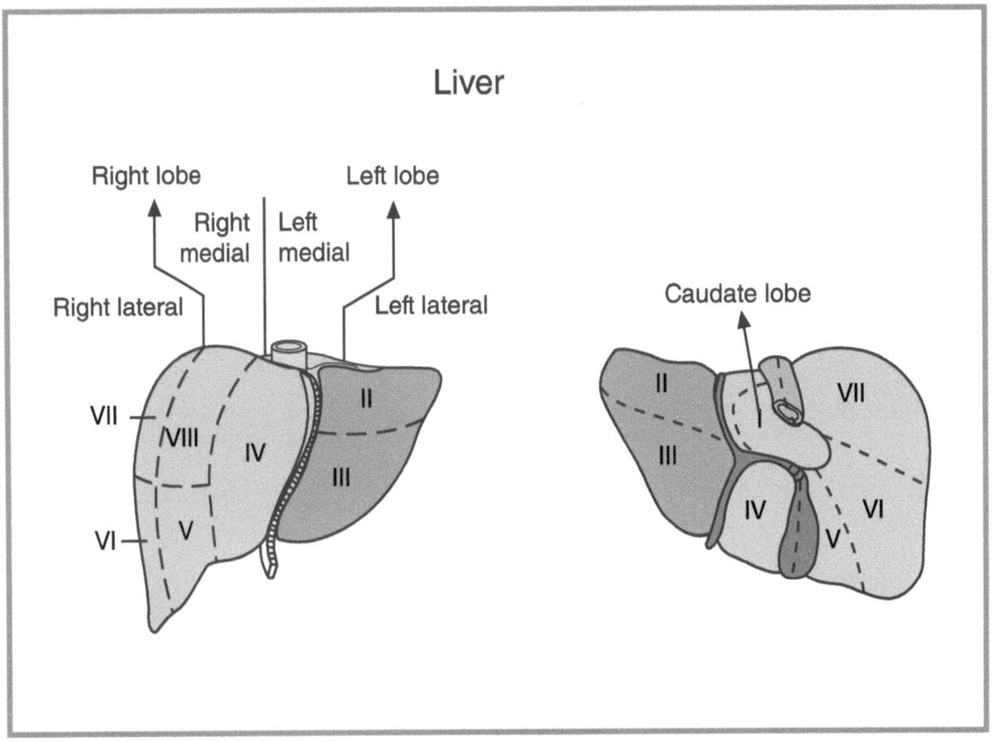

SEGMENTS OF THE LIVER

Segmental Liver Anatomy

Left lobe	Right lobe
I. Caudate (posterior) segment	V. Anterior medial (anterior inferior) segment
II. Lateral posterior (lateral superior) segment	VI. Anterior lateral (posterior inferior) segment
III. Lateral anterior (lateral interior) segment	VII. Posterior lateral (posterior superior) segment
IV. Medial (medial superior and inferior) segment	VIII. Posterior medial (anterior superior) segment

The labels above reflect the new International Anatomical Terminology. Previous terminology is in brackets.

References

1. Moore KL, Dalley AF. Clinically Oriented Anatomy. Fifth Ed., Lippincott Williams & Wilkins, Philadelphia. 2006, p: 294–295.
2. Skandalakis JE, Branum GD, Colborn GL, Mirilas P, Weidman TA, Skandalakis LJ, Kingsnorth AN, Skandalakis PN, Zoras O. Liver. In: Skandalakis JE (Ed. in Chief), Skandalakis' Surgical Anatomy. Vol. II, Ch. 19. Paschalidis Medical Publications, Athens. 2004, p: 1026–1036.
3. Borley NR, Toogood G. Hepatobiliary System: Liver. In: Standring S (Ed. in Chief), Gray's Anatomy. Ch. 85, Thirty-Ninth Ed., Elsevier Churchill-Livingstone, Edinburgh. 2005, p: 1216–1218.
4. Csillag A. Anatomy of the Living Human: Atlas of Medical Imaging. Könemann, Köln. 2000, p: 204–205.

Adapted and modified from Moore KL, et al.

* *Moore KL, Dalley AF. II. Clinically Oriented Anatomy. 4th ed. Philadelphia: Lippincott Williams & Wilkins, 1999.*

Picture 1

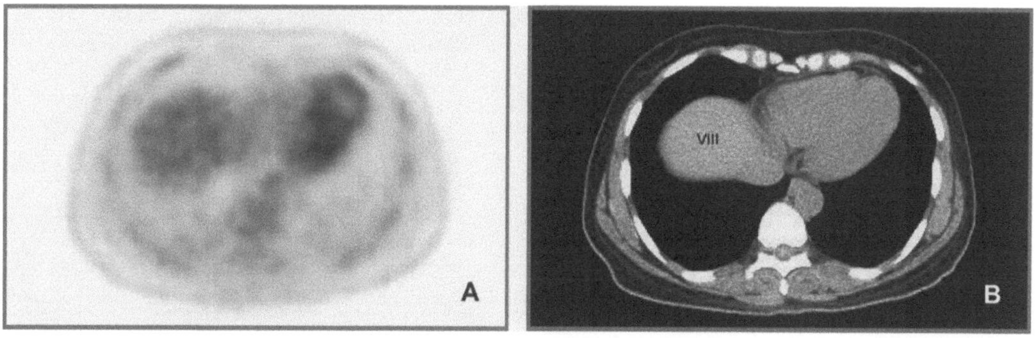

Picture 2

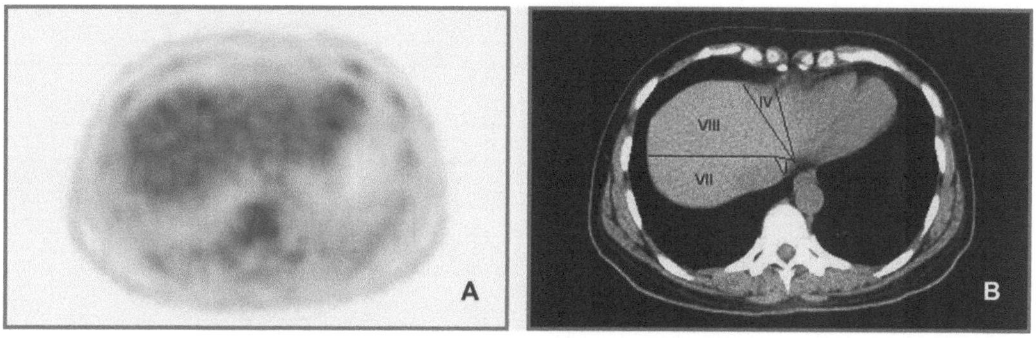

Picture 3

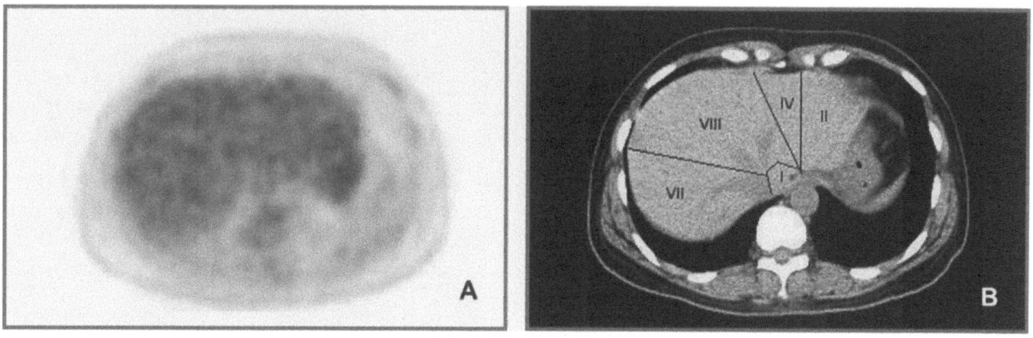

Keys

Left lobe	Right lobe
1. Caudate (posterior) segment	V. Anterior medial (anterior inferior) segment
II. Lateral posterior (lateral superior) segment	VI. Anterior lateral (posterior inferior) segment
III. Lateral anterior (lateral interior) segment	III. Posterior lateral (posterior superior) segment
IV. Medial (medial superior and inferior) segment	IV. Posterior medial (anterior superior) segment

Picture 4

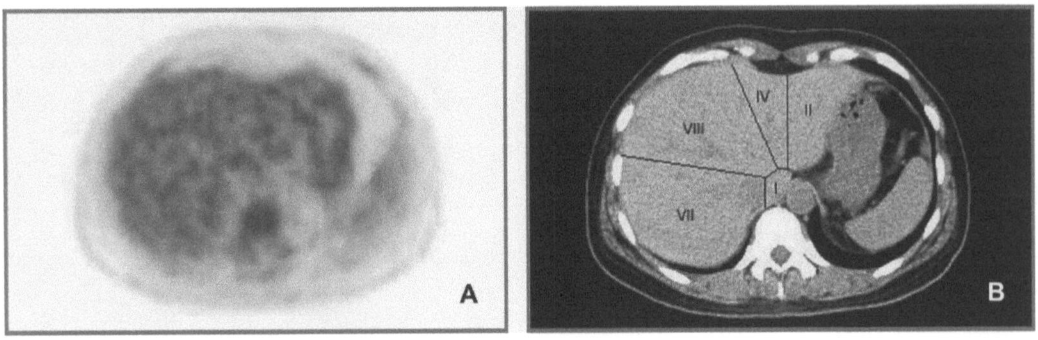

Picture 5

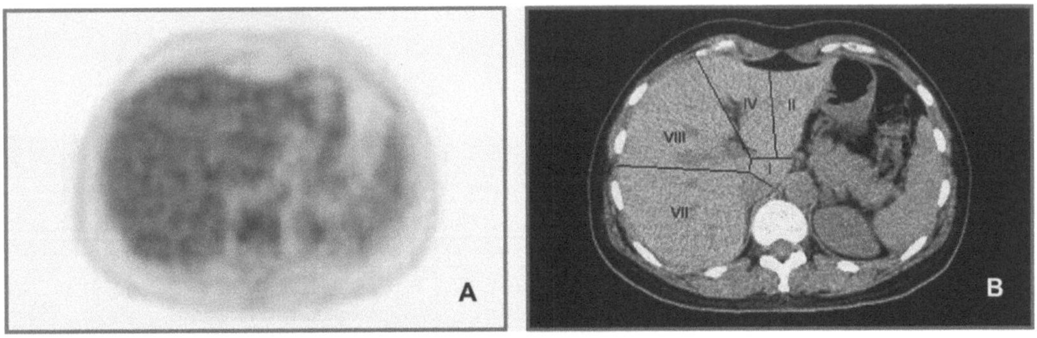

Picture 6

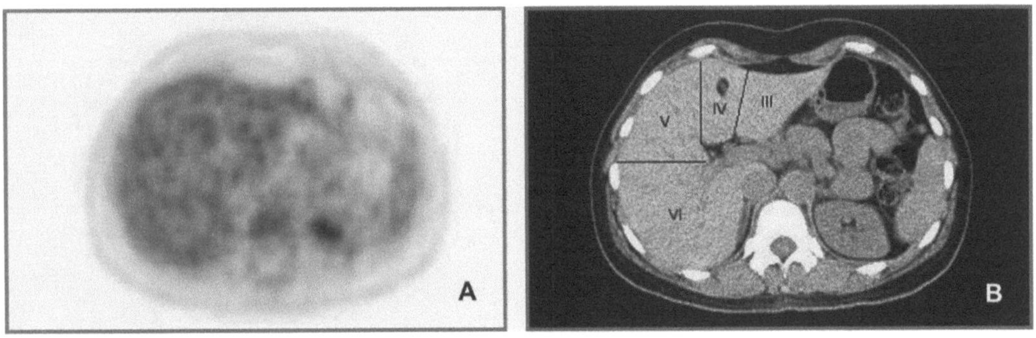

Keys

Left lobe

I. Caudate (posterior) segment
II. Lateral posterior (lateral superior) segment
III. Lateral anterior (lateral interior) segment
IV. Medial (medial superior and inferior) segment

Right lobe

V. Anterior medial (anterior inferior) segment
VI. Anterior lateral (posterior inferior) segment
VII. Posterior lateral (posterior superior) segment
VIII. Posterior medial (anterior superior) segment

Picture 7

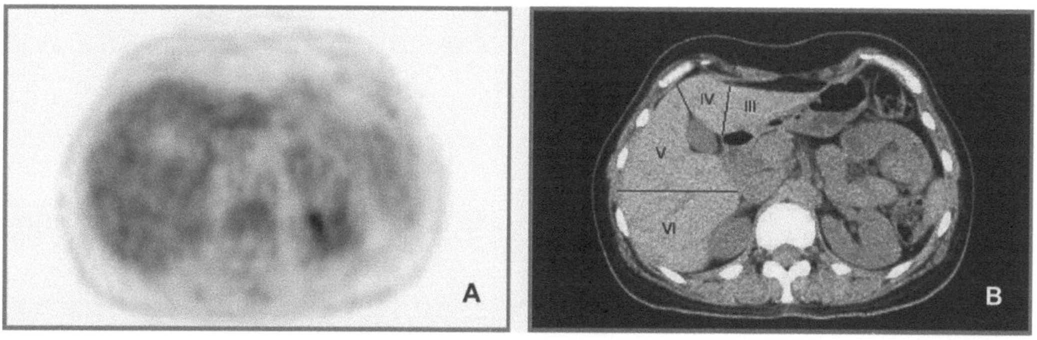

Picture 8

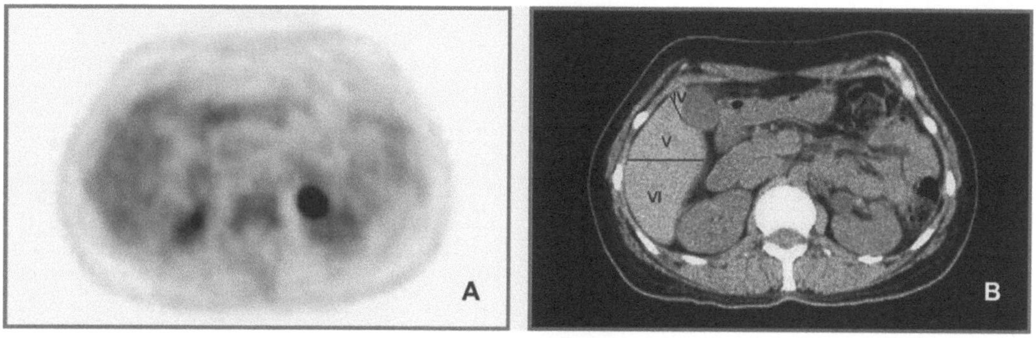

Picture 9

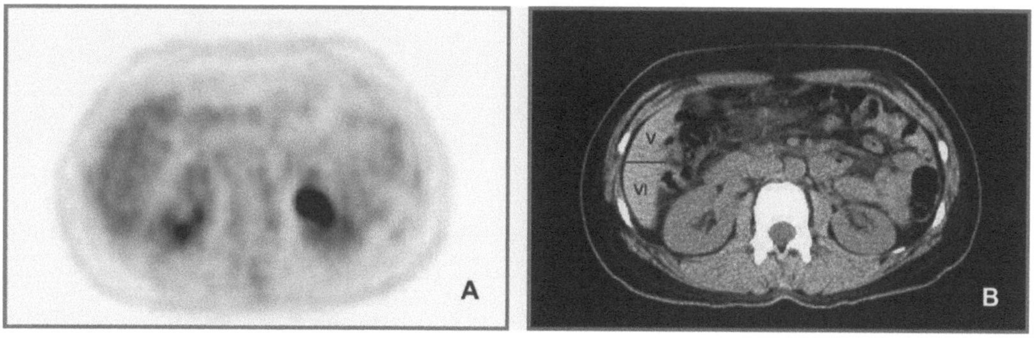

Keys

Left lobe	Right lobe
I. Caudate (posterior) segment	V. Anterior medial (anterior inferior) segment
II. Lateral posterior (lateral superior) segment	VI. Anterior lateral (posterior inferior) segment
III. Lateral anterior (lateral interior) segment	VII. Posterior lateral (posterior superior) segment
IV. Medial (medial superior and inferior) segment	VIII. Posterior medial (anterior superior) segment

Chapter 4
Pelvis

M.T. Kitapçı, *Atlas of Sectional Radiological Anatomy for PET/CT*,
DOI 10.1007/978-1-4614-1527-5_4, © Springer Science+Business Media New York 2012

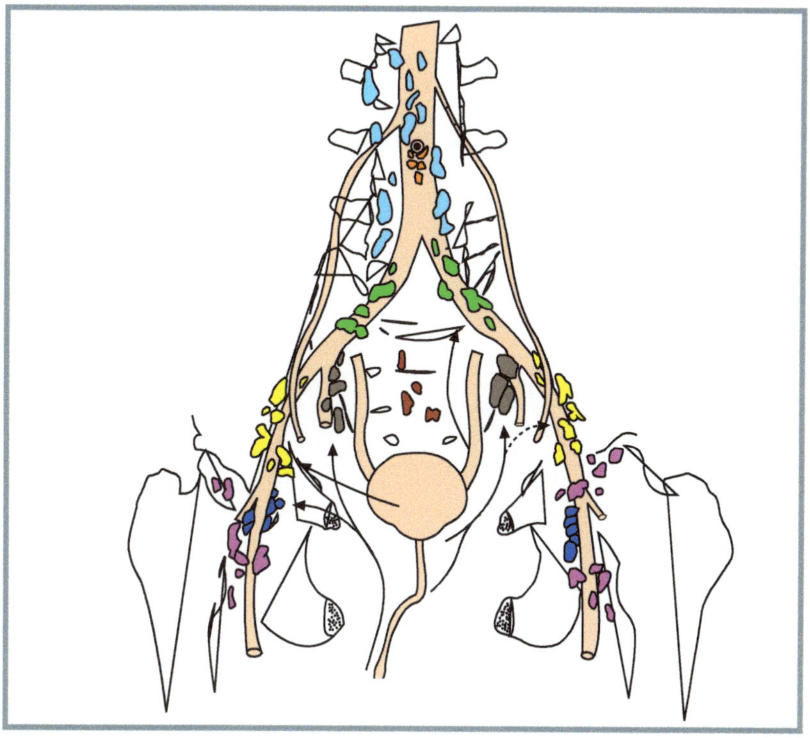

PELVIS

Lymph Nodes

Pelvis
Lateral aortic
Inferior mesenteric
Common iliac
Internal iliac
External iliac
Superficial inguinal
Deep inguinal
Sacral
Pararectal

Adapted and modified from Moore KL, et al.

* *Moore KL, Dalley AF. II. Clinically Oriented Anatomy. 4th ed. Philadelphia: Lippincott Williams & Wilkins, 1999.*

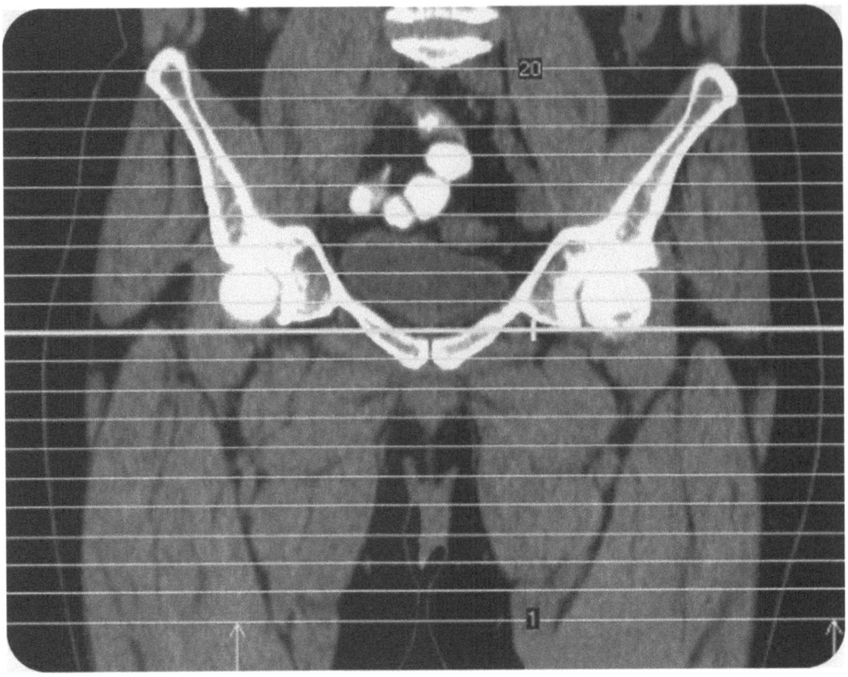

Consecutive sections were obtained with 3-mm slice thickness and without intravenous contrast. Positron Emission Tomography (PET) scintigraphic and Computed Tomography (CT) images obtained from the same level were given side to side for comparison. All anatomic structures in an image were numbered and given in the explanation section at the bottom of the page. Vertebral levels were marked on each vertebra.

Pelvis (Female)

Picture 1

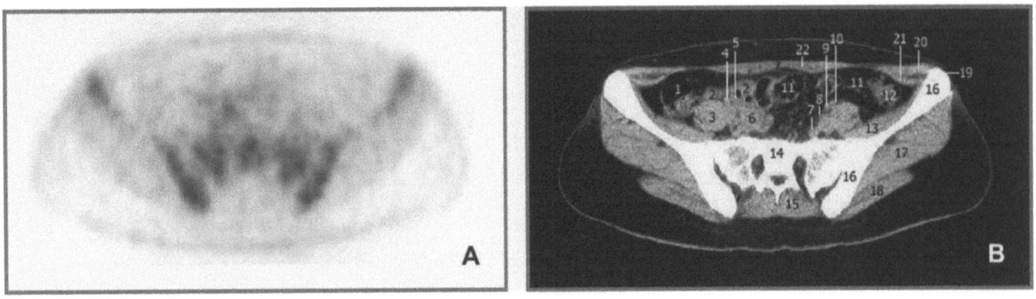

Picture 2

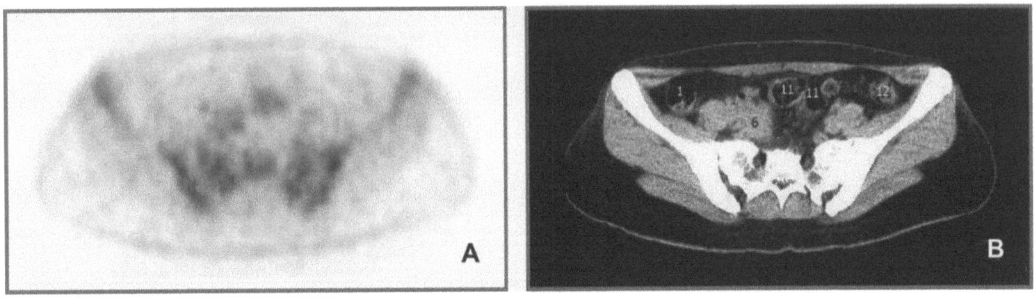

Picture 3

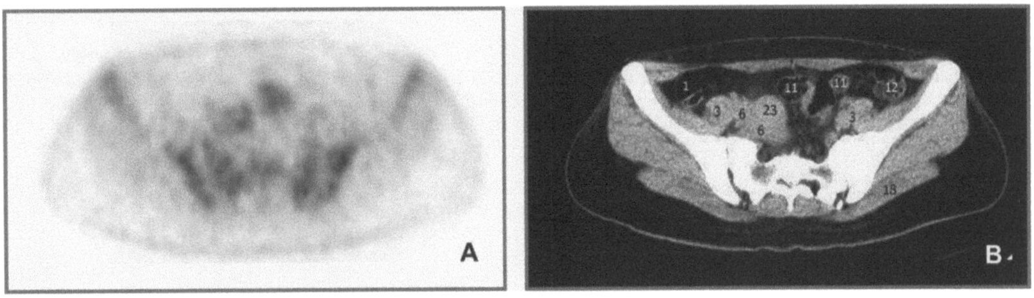

Keys

1. Caecum
2. Terminal ileum
3. Psoas major
4. Right external iliac artery
5. Right external iliac vein
6. Ileum
7. Left internal iliac vein
8. Left ureter
9. Left external iliac vein
10. Left external iliac artery
11. Sigmoid colon
12. Descending colon
13. Iliacus
14. Sacrum
15. Erector spinae
16. Wing of ilium
17. Gluteus medius
18. Gluteus maximus
19. Anterior superior iliac spine
20. Obliquus internus abdominis
21. Transversus abdominis
22. Rectus abdominis
23. Fundus uteri

Picture 4

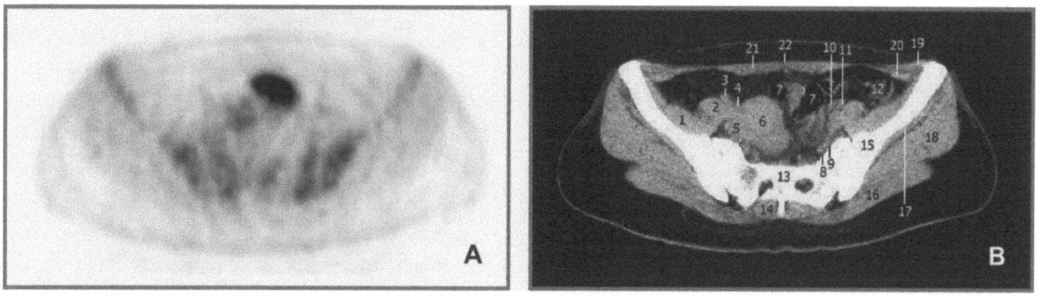

Picture 5

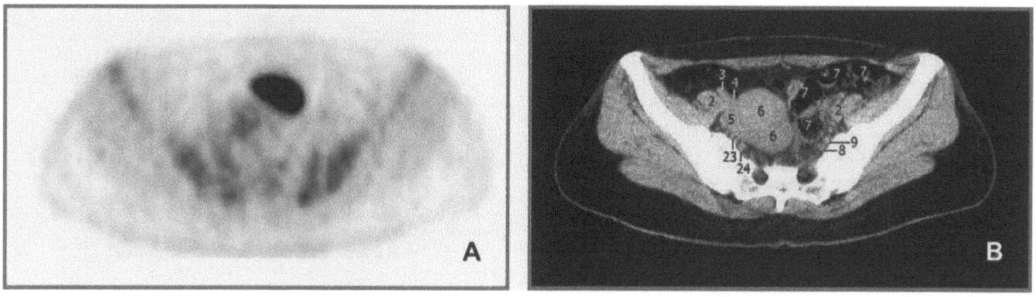

Picture 6

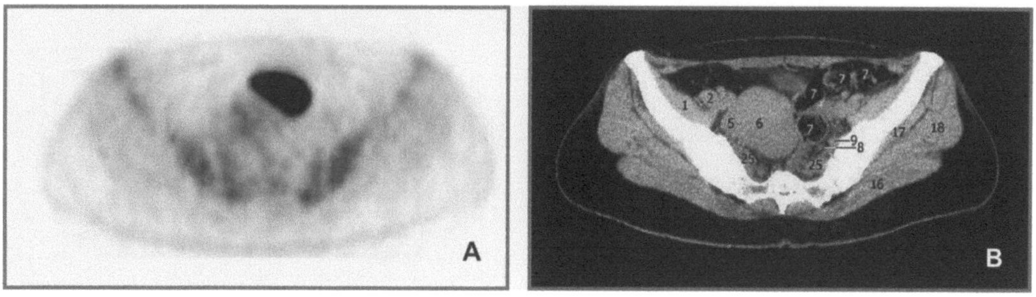

Keys

1. Iliacus
2. Psoas major
3. Right external iliac artery
4. Right external iliac vein
5. Right ovary
6. Fundus uteri
7. Sigmoid colon
8. Left internal iliac vein
9. Left internal iliac artery
10. Left external iliac vein
11. Left external iliac artery
12. Descending colon
13. Sacrum
14. Erector spinae
15. Iliac bone
16. Gluteus maximus
17. Gluteus minimus
18. Gluteus medius
19. Obliquus internus abdominis
20. Transversus abdominis
21. Rectus abdominis
22. Linea alba
23. Right internal iliac artery
24. Right internal iliac vein
25. Piriformis

Picture 7

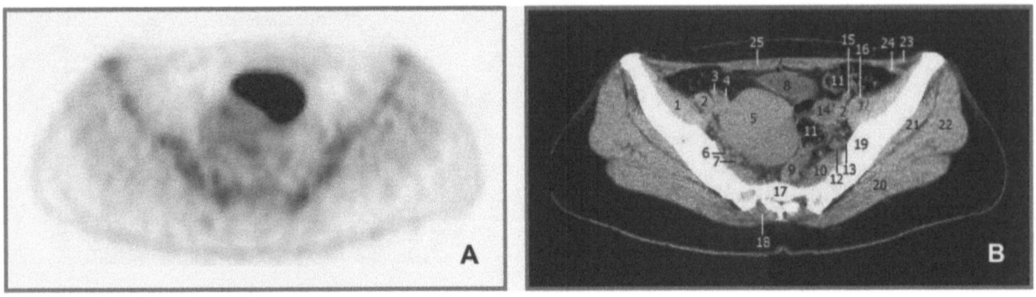

Picture 8

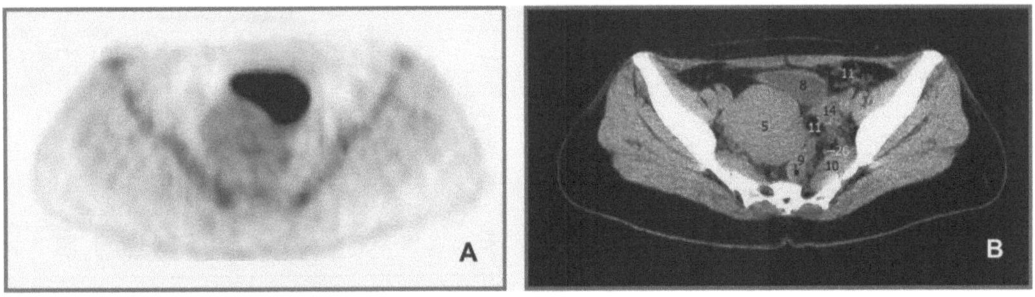

Picture 9

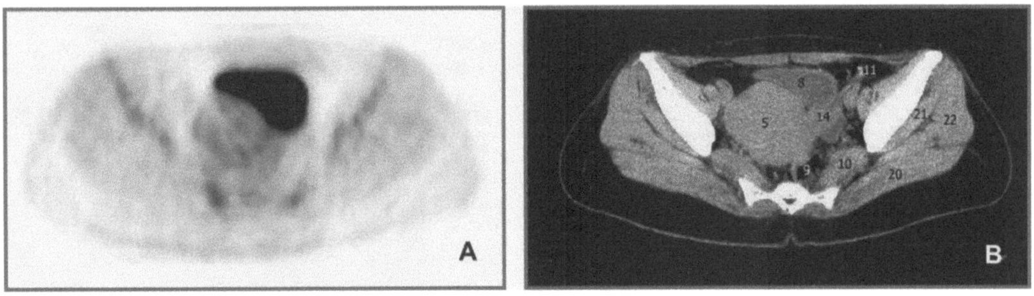

Keys

1. Iliacus
2. Psoas major
3. Right external iliac artery
4. Right external iliac vein
5. Corpus uteri
6. Right internal iliac artery
7. Right internal iliac vein
8. Urinary bladder
9. Rectosigmoid colon
10. Piriformis
11. Sigmoid colon
12. Left internal iliac vein
13. Left internal iliac artery
14. Left ovary
15. Left external iliac vein
16. Left external iliac artery
17. Sacrum
18. Erector spinae
19. Iliac bone
20. Gluteus maximus
21. Gluteus minimus
22. Gluteus medius
23. Obliquus internus abdominis
24. Transversus abdominis
25. Rectus abdominis
26. Sciatic nerve

Picture 10

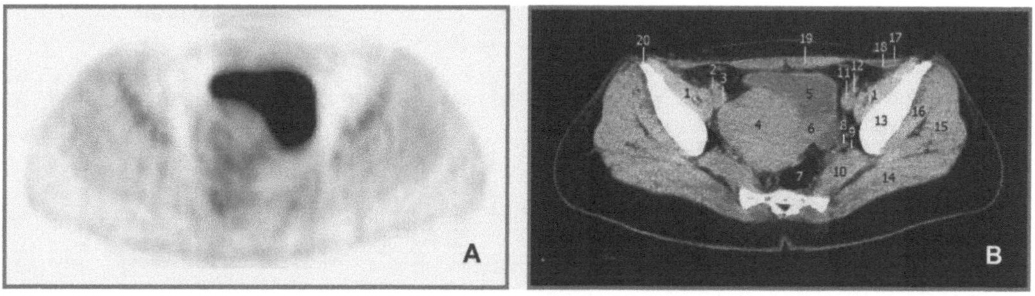

Picture 11

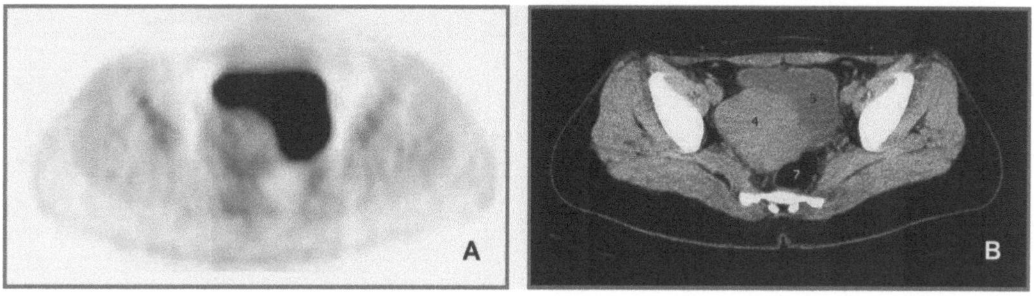

Picture 12

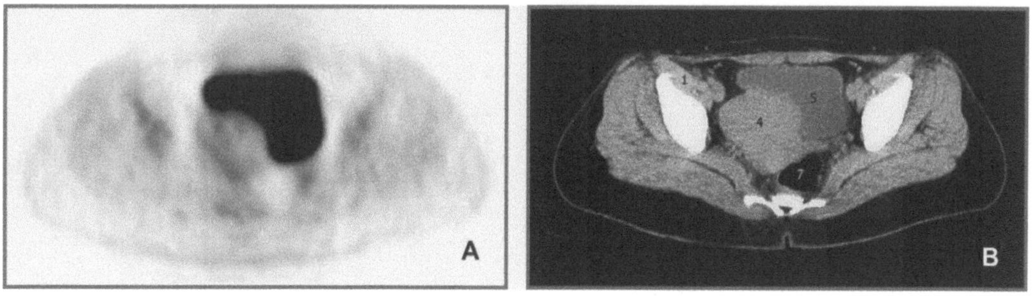

Keys

1. Iliopsoas
2. Right external iliac artery
3. Right external iliac vein
4. Corpus uteri
5. Urinary bladder
6. Left ovary
7. Rectum
8. Left internal iliac vein
9. Left internal iliac artery
10. Piriformis
11. Left external iliac vein
12. Left external iliac artery
13. Iliac bone
14. Gluteus maximus
15. Gluteus medius
16. Gluteus minimus
17. Obliquus internus abdominis
18. Transversus abdominis
19. Rectus abdominis
20. Anterior inferior iliac spine

Picture 13

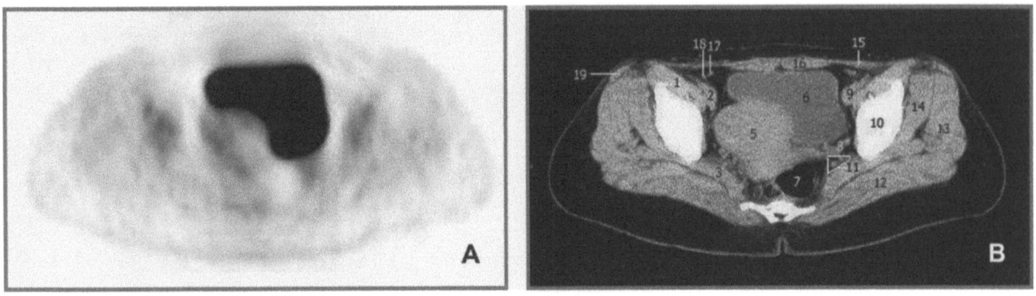

Picture 14

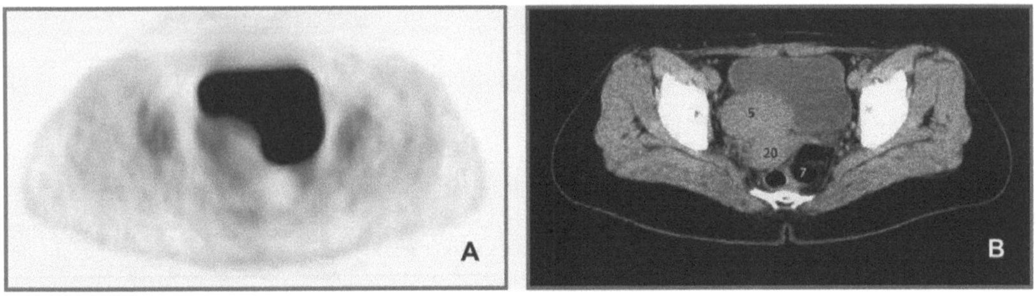

Picture 15

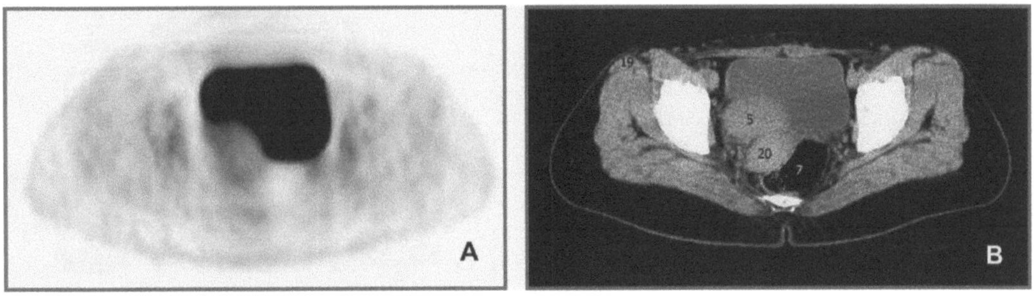

Keys

1. Iliopsoas
2. Right external iliac artery and vein
3. Piriformis
4. Right internal iliac artery and vein
5. Corpus uteri
6. Urinary bladder
7. Rectum
8. Left internal iliac artery and vein
9. Left external iliac artery and vein
10. Ischium
11. Sacral plexus
12. Gluteus maximus
13. Gluteus medius
14. Gluteus minimus
15. Obliquus internus abdominis (aponeurosis)
16. Rectus abdominis
17. Inferior epigastric artery and vein
18. Round ligament of uterus
19. Tensor fasciae latae
20. Cervix uteri

Picture 16

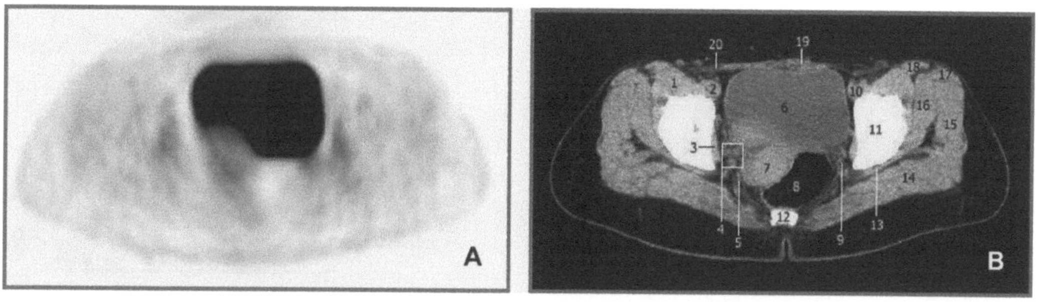

Picture 17

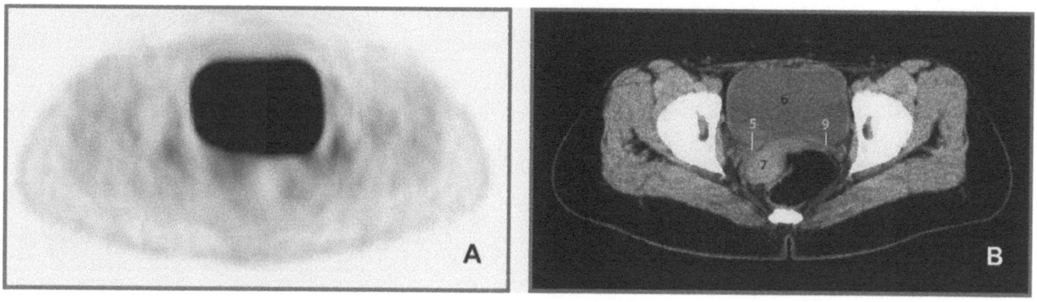

Picture 18

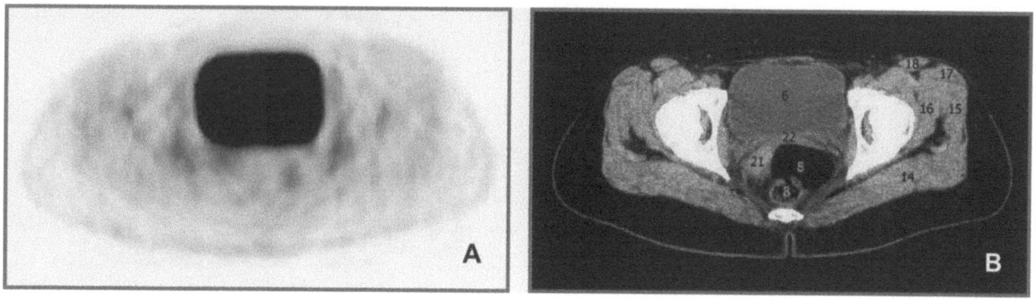

Keys

1. Iliopsoas
2. Right external iliac artery and vein
3. Obturatorius internus
4. Right internal iliac artery and vein
5. Right ureter
6. Urinary bladder
7. Cervix uteri
8. Rectum
9. Left ureter
10. Left external iliac artery and vein
11. Ischium
12. Coccyx
13. Piriformis (tendon)
14. Gluteus maximus
15. Gluteus medius
16. Gluteus minimus
17. Tensor fasciae latae
18. Sartorius
19. Rectus abdominis
20. Obliquus internus abdominis (aponeurosis)
21. Cervix uteri (vaginal part)
22. Vagina

Picture 19

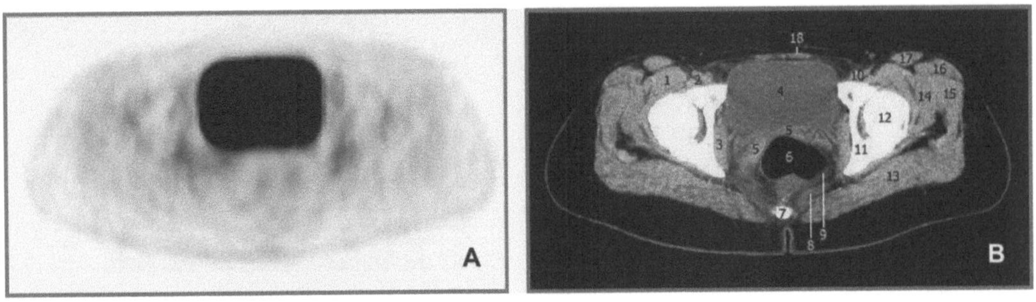

Picture 20

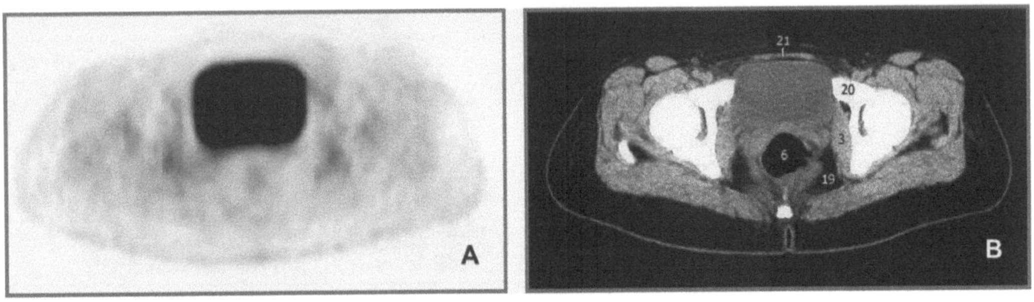

Picture 21

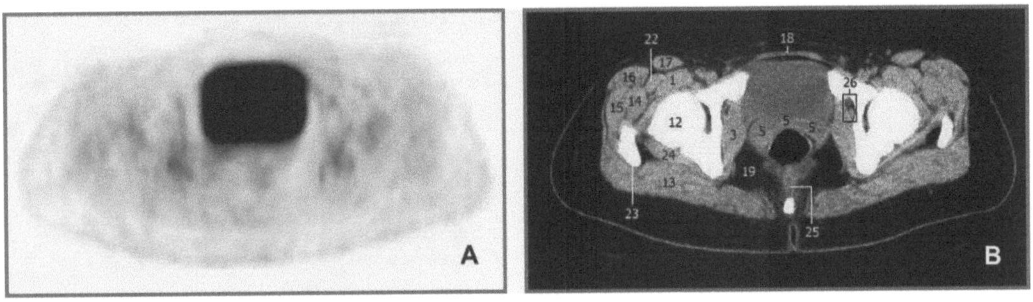

Keys

1. Iliopsoas
2. Right external iliac artery and vein
3. Obturatorius internus
4. Urinary bladder
5. Vagina
6. Rectum
7. Coccyx
8. Coccygeus
9. Levator ani
10. Left external iliac artery and vein
11. Acetabulum (ischium)
12. Head of femur
13. Gluteus maximus
14. Gluteus minimus
15. Gluteus medius
16. Tensor fasciae latae
17. Sartorius
18. Rectus abdominis (aponeurosis)
19. Ischiorectal fossa
20. Superior ramus of pubis
21. Pyramidalis
22. Rectus femoris
23. Femur, greater trochanter
24. Gemellus superior
25. Anococcygeal ligament
26. Obturator artery, vein and nerve

Picture 22

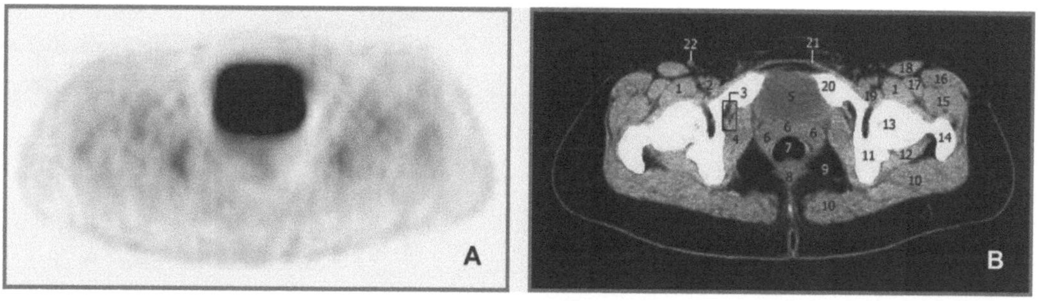

Picture 23

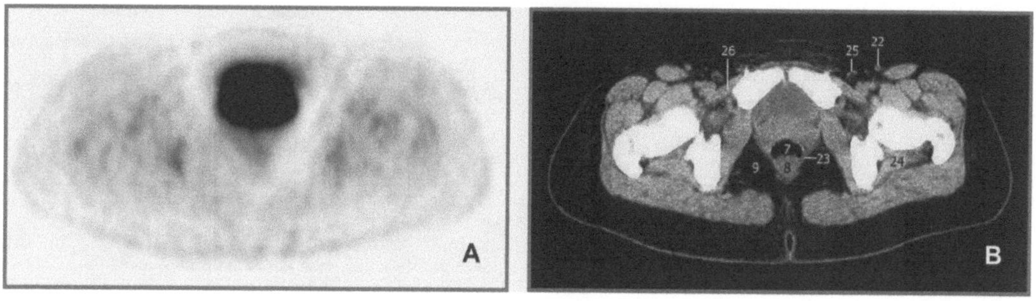

Picture 24

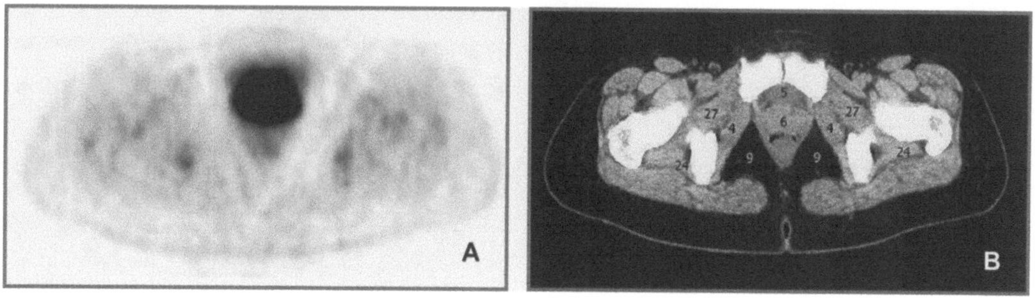

Keys

1. Iliopsoas
2. Right femoral artery and vein
3. Obturator artery, vein and nerve
4. Obturatorius internus
5. Urinary bladder
6. Vagina
7. Rectum
8. Anococcygeal ligament
9. Ischiorectal fossa
10. Gluteus maximus
11. Ischium
12. Gemellus superior
13. Head of femur
14. Femur, greater trochanter
15. Gluteus minimus and medius
16. Tensor fasciae latae
17. Rectus femoris
18. Sartorius
19. Left femoral artery and vein
20. Superior ramus of pubis
21. Inguinal ligament
22. Superficial circumflex iliac artery and vein
23. Levator ani
24. Gemellus inferior
25. Superficial epigastric artery and vein
26. Pectineus
27. Obturatorius externus

Picture 25

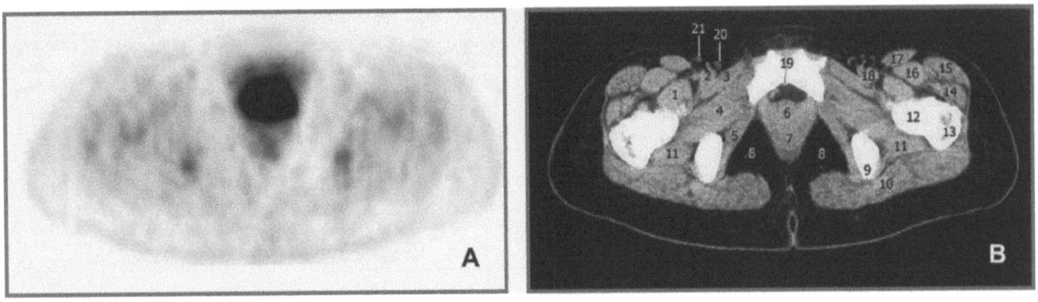

Picture 26

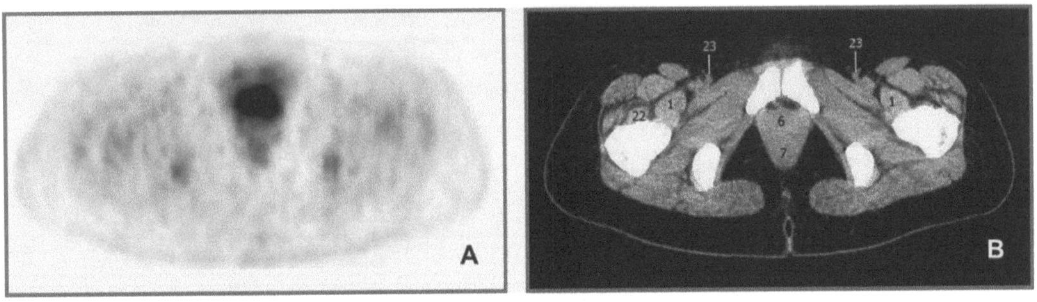

Picture 27

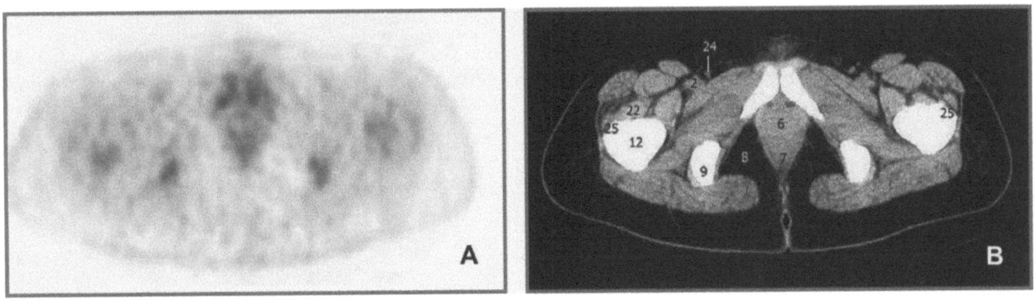

Keys

1. Iliopsoas
2. Right femoral artery and vein
3. Pectineus
4. Obturatorius externus
5. Obturatorius internus
6. Vagina
7. Anal canal
8. Ischiorectal fossa
9. Ischial tuberosity
10. Gluteus maximus
11. Quadratus femoris
12. Neck of femur
13. Femur, greater trochanter
14. Gluteus minimus and medius
15. Tensor fasciae latae
16. Rectus femoris
17. Sartorius
18. Left femoral artery and vein
19. Symphysis pubis
20. Superficial epigastric artery and vein
21. Superficial circumflex iliac artery and vein
22. Quadriceps femoris, vastus lateralis
23. Saphenous opening
24. Greater saphenous vein
25. Femur, lesser trochanter

Picture 28

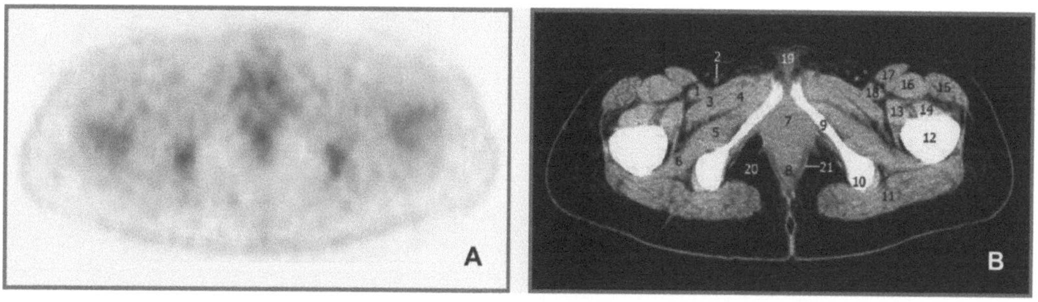

Picture 29

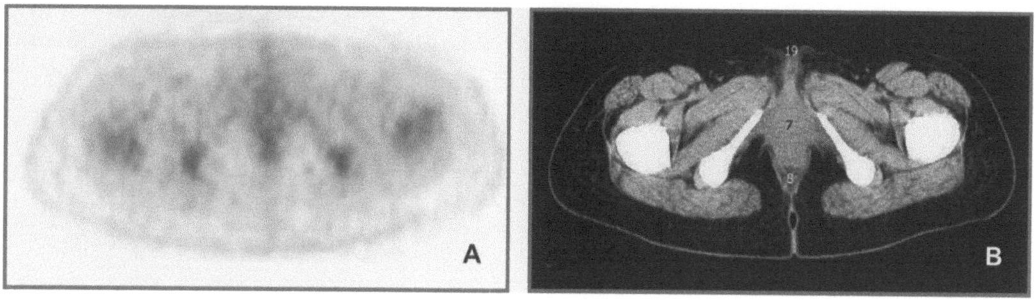

Keys

1. Right femoral artery and vein
2. Greater saphenous vein
3. Pectineus
4. Adductor brevis
5. Obturatorius externus
6. Quadratus femoris
7. Vagina
8. Anal canal
9. Inferior ramus of pubis
10. Ischial tuberosity
11. Gluteus maximus
12. Neck of femur
13. Iliopsoas
14. Quadriceps femoris, vastus lateralis
15. Tensor fasciae latae
16. Rectus femoris
17. Sartorius
18. Left femoral artery and vein
19. Rima pudendi
20. Ishiorectal fossa
21. Levator ani

Pelvis (Male)

Picture 1

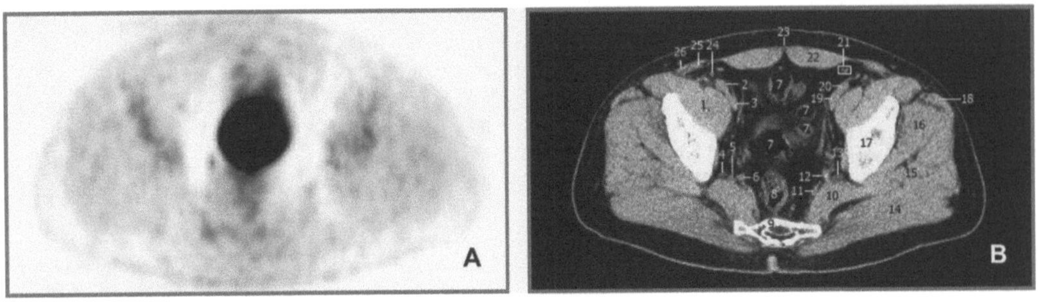

Picture 2

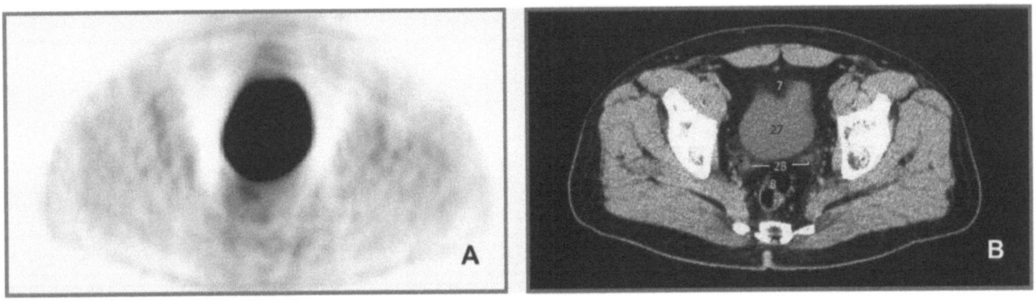

Picture 3

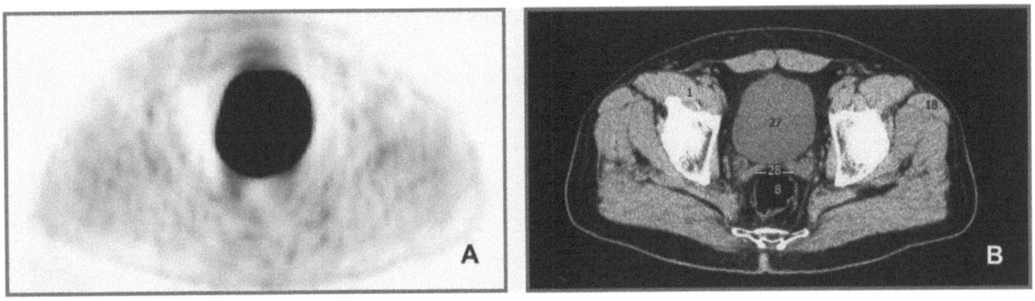

Keys

1. Iliopsoas
2. Right external iliac artery
3. Right external iliac vein
4. Right ureter
5. Right internal iliac artery
6. Right internal iliac vein
7. Sigmoid colon
8. Rectum
9. Sacral vertebra
10. Piriformis
11. Left internal iliac vein
12. Left internal iliac artery
13. Left ureter
14. Gluteus maximus
15. Gluteus medius
16. Gluteus minimus
17. Ischium
18. Tensor fasciae latae
19. Left external iliac vein
20. Left external iliac artery
21. Inferior epigastric artery and vein
22. Rectus abdominis
23. Linea alba
24. Ductus deferens
25. Transversus abdominis
26. Obliquus internus abdominis
27. Urinary bladder
28. Seminal vesicle

Picture 4

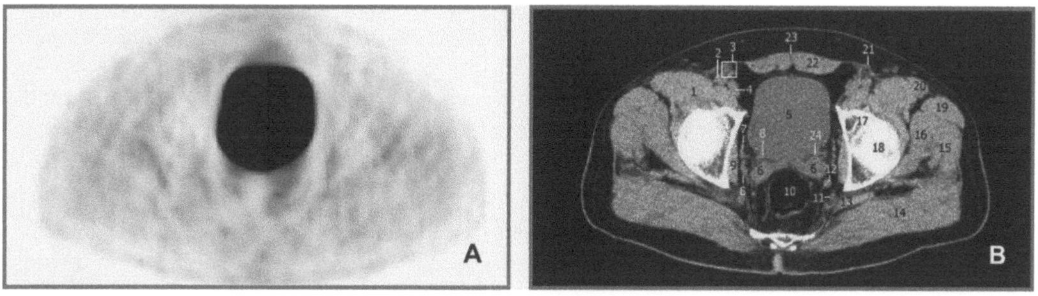

Picture 5

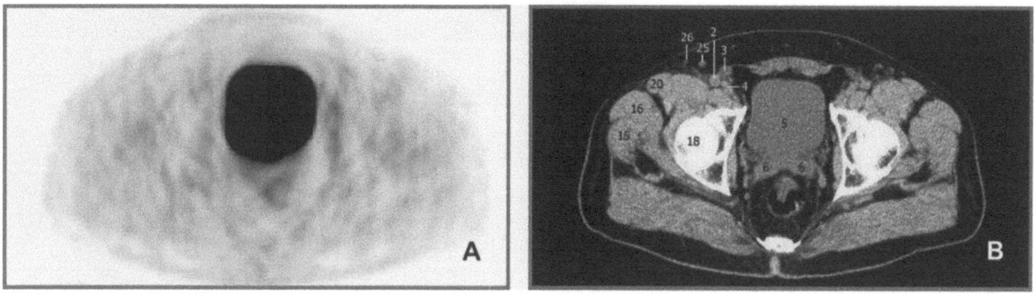

Picture 6

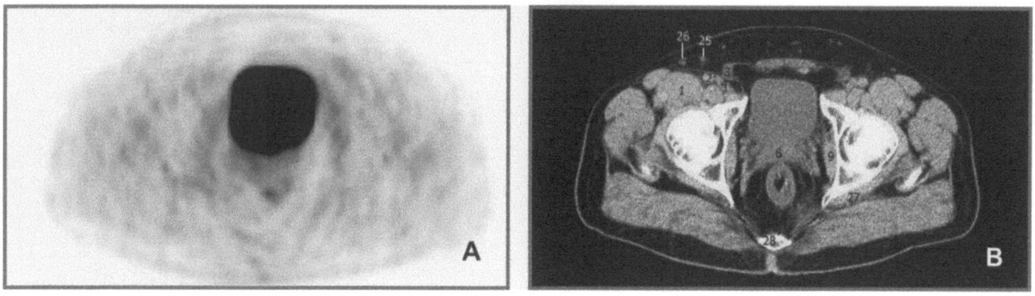

Keys

1. Iliopsoas
2. Right external iliac artery
3. Spermatic cord
4. Right external iliac vein
5. Urinary bladder
6. Seminal vesicle
7. Ductus deferens
8. Right ureter
9. Obturatorius internus
10. Rectum
11. Left sciatic nerve
12. Left internal iliac artery
13. Gemellus superior
14. Gluteus maximus
15. Gluteus medius
16. Gluteus minimus
17. Acetabulum (ischial bone)
18. Head of femur
19. Tensor fasciae latae
20. Sartorius
21. Inguinal ligament
22. Rectus abdominis
23. Linea alba
24. Left ureter
25. Superficial epigastric artery and vein
26. Superficial circumflex iliac artery and vein
27. Gemellus inferior
28. Coccyx

Picture 7

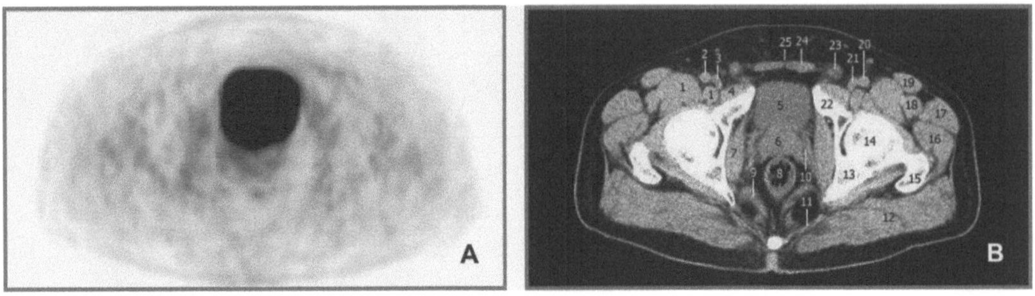

Picture 8

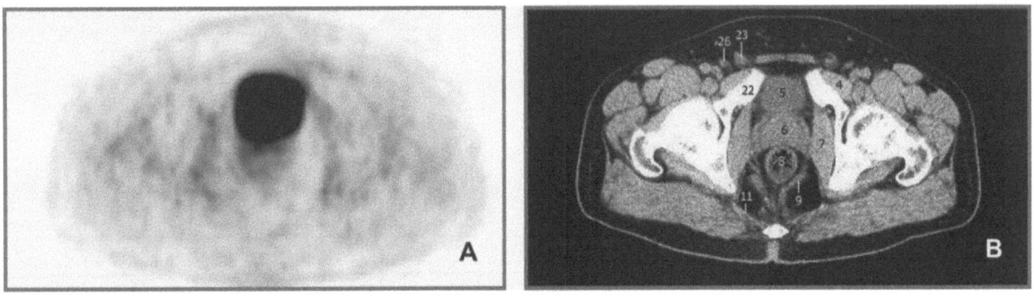

Picture 9

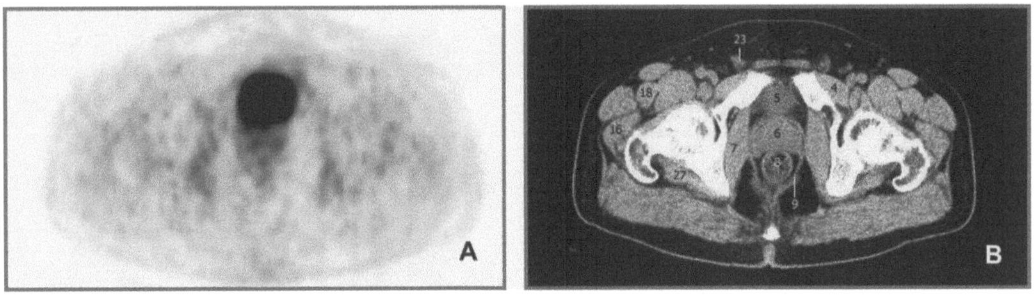

Keys

1. Iliopsoas
2. Right femoral artery
3. Right femoral vein
4. Pectineus
5. Urinary bladder
6. Prostate
7. Obturatorius internus
8. Rectum
9. Levator ani
10. Prostatic venous plexus
11. Coccygeus
12. Gluteus maximus
13. Ischium
14. Head of femur
15. Femur, greater trochanter
16. Gluteus medius and minimus
17. Tensor fasciae latae
18. Rectus femoris
19. Sartorius
20. Left femoral artery
21. Left femoral vein
22. Superior ramus of pubis
23. Spermatic cord
24. Rectus abdominis
25. Linea alba
26. Superficial inguinal lymph node
27. Quadratus femoris

Picture 10

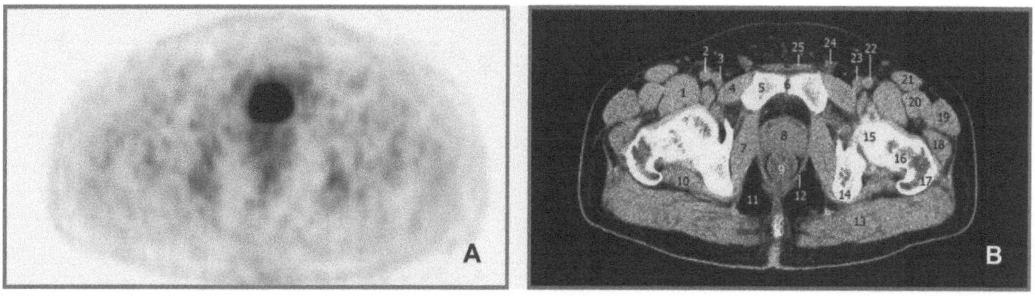

Picture 11

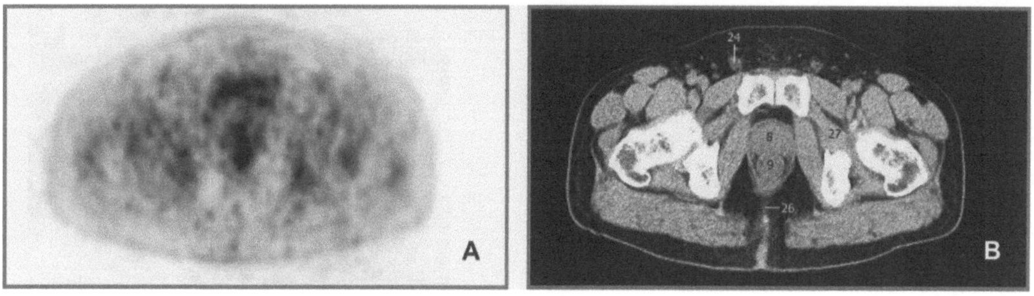

Picture 12

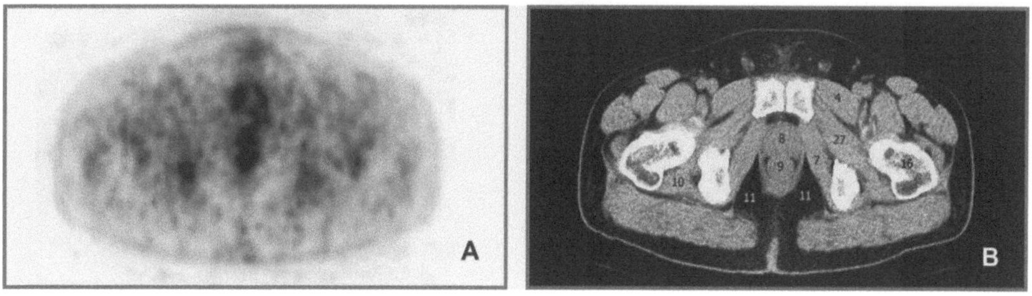

Keys

1. Iliopsoas
2. Right femoral artery
3. Right femoral vein
4. Pectineus
5. Superior ramus of pubis
6. Symphysis pubica
7. Obturatorius internus
8. Prostate
9. Anal canal
10. Quadratus femoris
11. Ischiorectal fossa
12. Levator ani
13. Gluteus maximus
14. Ischial tuberosity
15. Head of femur
16. Neck of femur
17. Femur, greater trochanter
18. Gluteus medius and minimus
19. Tensor fasciae latae
20. Rectus femoris
21. Sartorius
22. Left femoral artery
23. Left femoral vein
24. Spermatic cord
25. Rectus abdominis
26. Anococcygeal ligament
27. Obturatorius externus

Picture 13

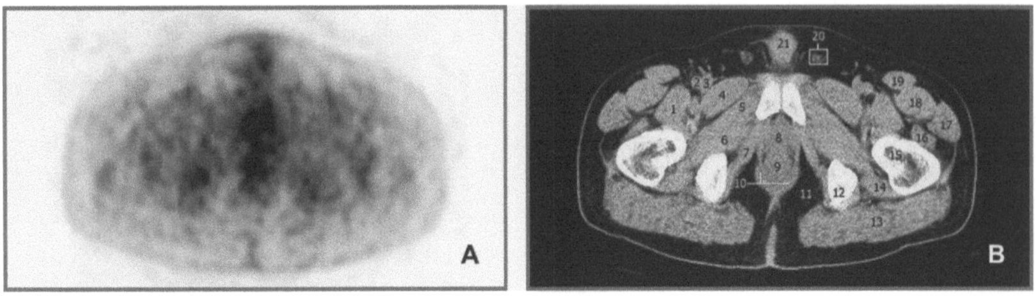

Picture 14

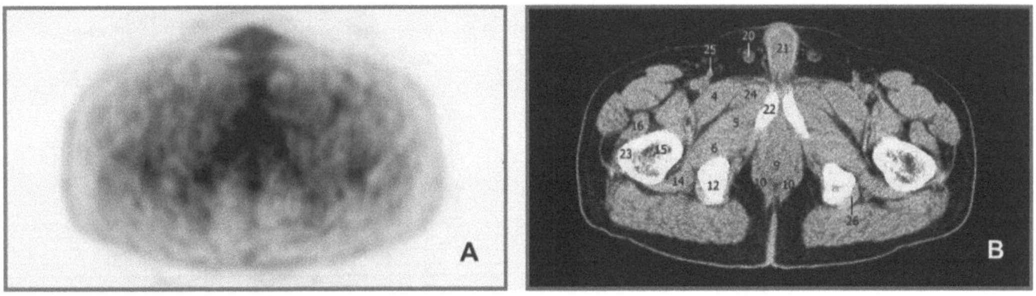

Picture 15

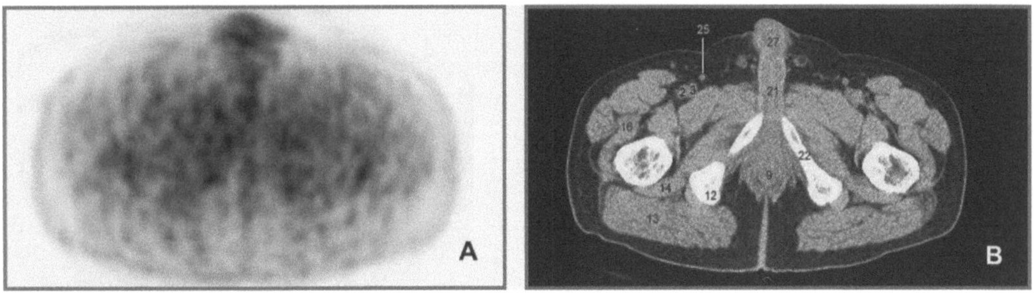

Keys

1. Iliopsoas
2. Femoral artery
3. Femoral vein
4. Pectineus
5. Adductor brevis
6. Obturatorius externus
7. Obturatorius internus
8. Prostate
9. Anal canal
10. Puborectalis
11. Ischiorectal fossa
12. Ischial tuberosity
13. Gluteus maximus
14. Quadratus femoris
15. Neck of femur
16. Quadriceps femoris, vastus lateralis
17. Tensor fasciae latae
18. Rectus femoris
19. Sartorius
20. Spermatic cord
21. Root of penis
22. Inferior ramus of pubis
23. Femur, lesser trochanter
24. Adductor longus
25. Greater saphenous vein
26. Long head of biceps femoris
27. Body of penis

Picture 16

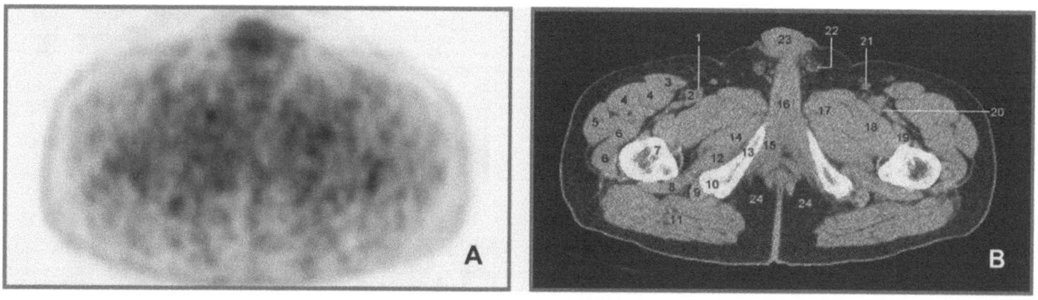

Picture 17

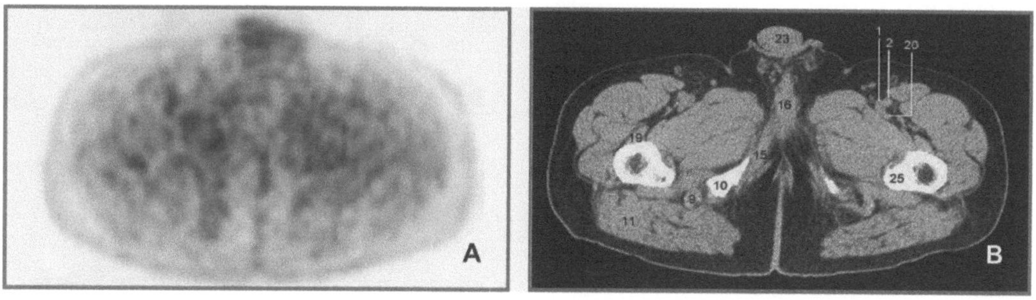

Picture 18

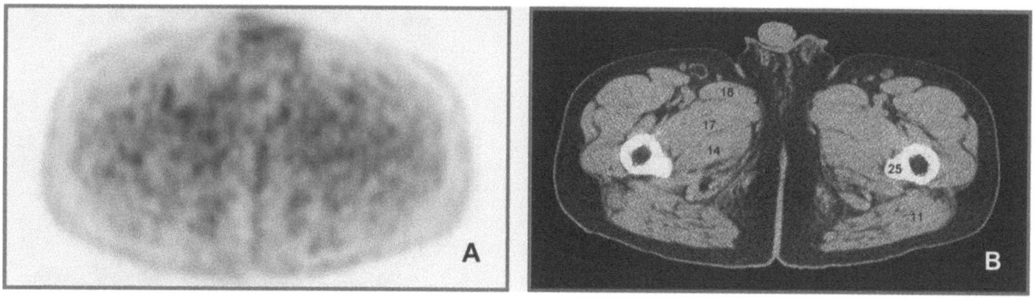

Keys

1. Femoral vein
2. Femoral artery
3. Sartorius
4. Rectus femoris
5. Tensor fasciae latae
6. Quadriceps femoris, vastus lateralis
7. Neck of femur
8. Quadratus femoris
9. Long head of biceps femoris
10. Ischial tuberosity
11. Gluteus maximus
12. Obturatorius externus
13. Inferior ramus of pubis
14. Adductor magnus
15. Crus of penis
16. Root of penis
17. Adductor brevis
18. Adductor longus
19. Pectineus
20. Femoral nerve
21. Greater saphenous vein
22. Spermatic cord
23. Body of penis
24. Ischiorectal fossa
25. Femur, lesser trochanter

Picture 19

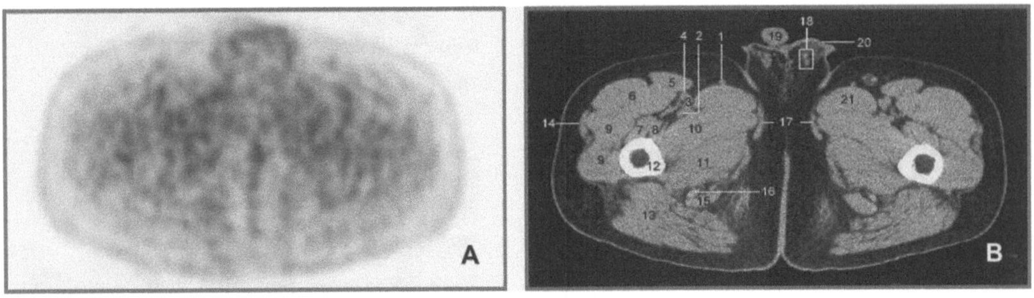

Picture 20

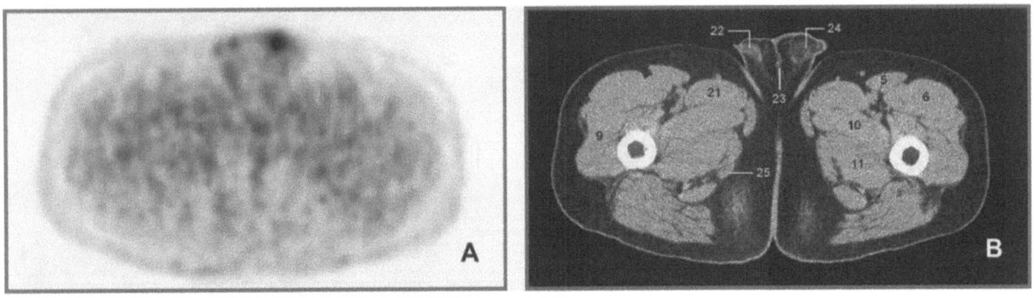

Picture 21

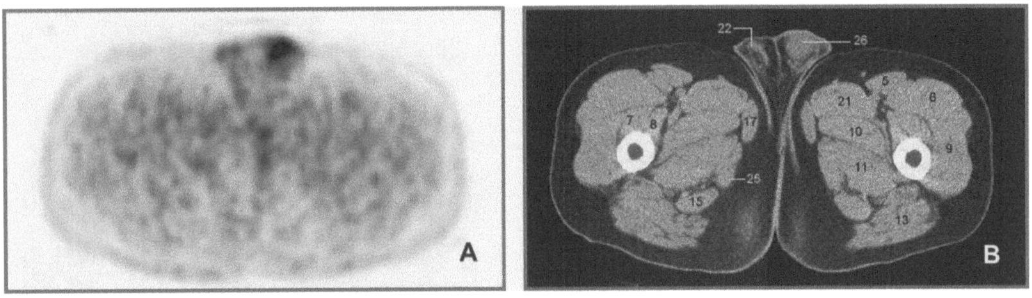

Keys

1. Greater saphenous vein
2. Femoral nerve
3. Femoral vein
4. Femoral artery
5. Sartorius
6. Rectus femoris
7. Quadriceps femoris, vastus intermedius
8. Quadriceps femoris, vastus medialis
9. Quadriceps femoris, vastus lateralis
10. Adductor brevis
11. Adductor magnus
12. Femur
13. Gluteus maximus
14. Tensor fasciae latae
15. Biceps femoris and semitendinosus
16. Sciatic nerve
17. Gracilis
18. Spermatic cord (in the scrotum)
19. Glans penis
20. Scrotum
21. Adductor longus
22. Right head of epididymis
23. Septum of scrotum
24. Left head of epididymis
25. Semimembranosus
26. Left testis

Picture 22

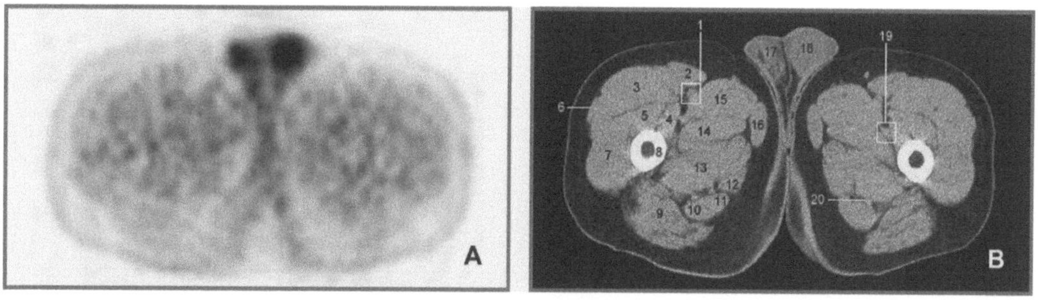

Picture 23

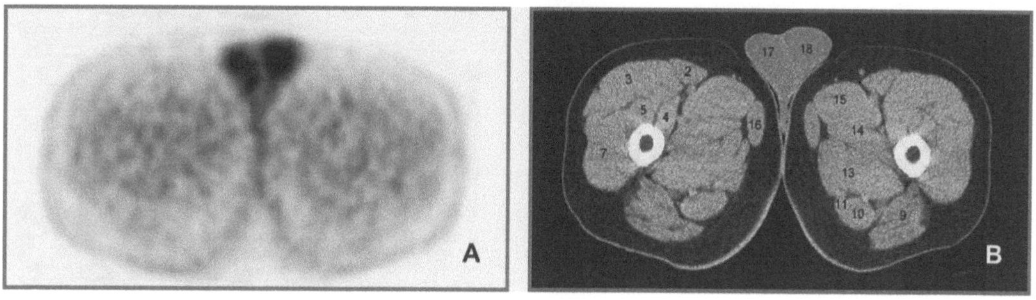

Picture 24

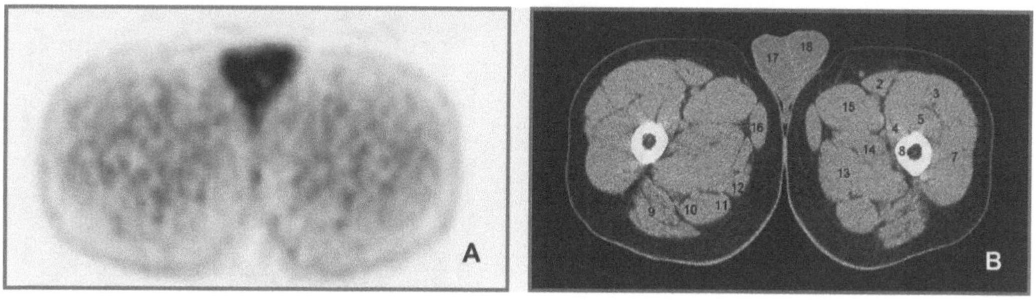

Keys

1. Femoral artery, vein and nerve
2. Sartorius
3. Rectus femoris
4. Quadriceps femoris, vastus medialis
5. Quadriceps femoris, vastus intermedius
6. Tensor fasciae latae
7. Quadriceps femoris, vastus lateralis
8. Femur
9. Gluteus maximus
10. Long head of biceps femoris
11. Semitendinosus
12. Semimembranosus
13. Adductor magnus
14. Adductor brevis
15. Adductor longus
16. Gracilis
17. Right testis
18. Left testis
19. Deep femoral artery and vein
20. Sciatic nerve

Picture 25

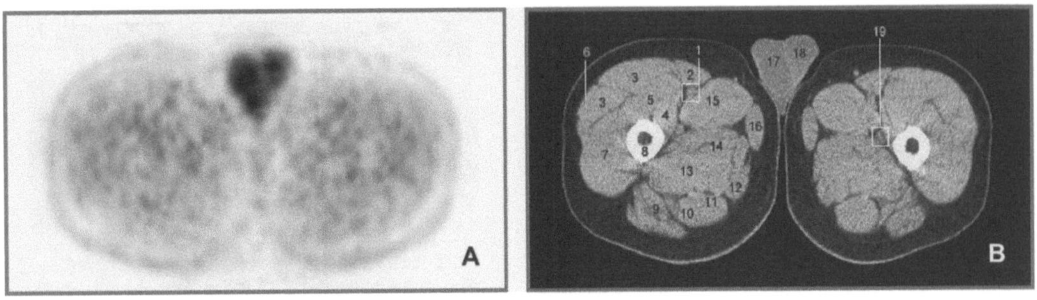

Picture 26

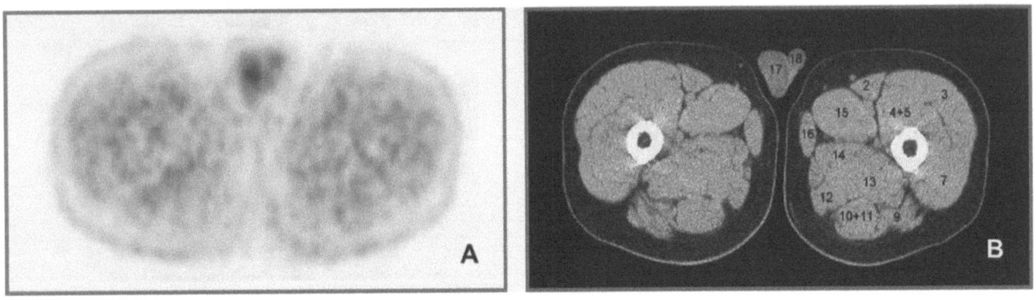

Picture 27

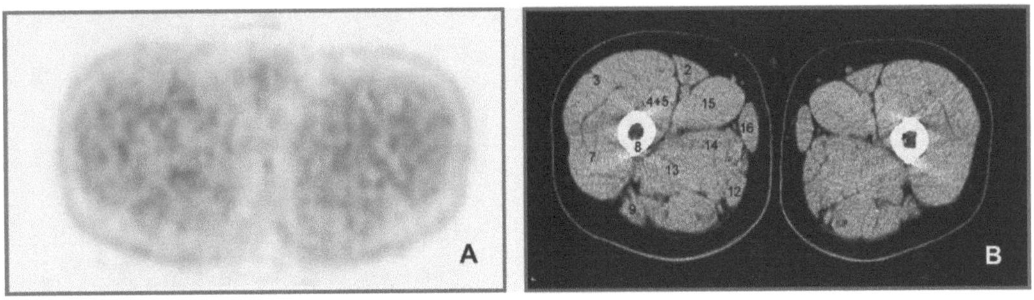

Keys

1. Femoral artery and vein
2. Sartorius
3. Rectus femoris
4. Quadriceps femoris, vastus medialis
5. Quadriceps femoris, vastus intermedius
6. Tensor fasciae latae
7. Quadriceps femoris, vastus lateralis
8. Femur
9. Gluteus maximus
10. Long head of biceps femoris
11. Semitendinosus
12. Semimembranosus
13. Adductor magnus
14. Adductor brevis
15. Adductor longus
16. Gracilis
17. Right testis
18. Left testis
19. Deep femoral artery and vein

Index

M.T. Kitapçı, *Atlas of Sectional Radiological Anatomy for PET/CT*,
DOI 10.1007/978-1-4614-1527-5, © Springer Science+Business Media New York 2012

FSC
www.fsc.org
MIX
Papier | Fördert gute Waldnutzung
FSC® C083411

Kolibri 360 GmbH
Ferdinand-Jühlke-Straße 7
99095 Erfurt, Deutschland
produktsicherheit@kolibri360.de